Other Times, Other Realities

Other Times, Other Realities

Toward a Theory of Psychoanalytic Treatment

Arnold H. Modell

Harvard University Press
Cambridge, Massachusetts
London, England
1990

Excerpts from "Burnt Norton" in *Four Quartets* by T. S. Eliot, copyright 1943
by T. S. Eliot and renewed 1971 by Esme Valerie Eliot, are reprinted by
permission of Harcourt Brace Jovanovich, Inc., and of Faber and Faber Ltd.

This book is printed on acid-free paper, and its binding materials
have been chosen for strength and durability.

Library of Congress Cataloging-in-Publication Data
Modell, Arnold H., 1924–
   Other times, other realities : toward a theory of psychoanalytic
treatment / Arnold H. Modell.
       p.   cm.
   Includes bibliographical references.
   ISBN 0-674-64498-0 (alk. paper)
   1. Psychoanalysis. I. Title.
   [DNLM: 1. Psychoanalytic Theory. 2. Psychoanalytic Therapy. WM
460 M689oa]
RC506.M63   1990
616.89'17—dc20
DNLM/DLC   89-19967
for Library of Congress   CIP

For Naomi, Bess, Oscar, and Mukunda

Acknowledgments

I am grateful to my patients, who have been my unwitting collaborators; without them I could not have written this book. I am also indebted to my students at the Beth Israel Hospital, who responded to the work in progress.

I am especially grateful to my friends and colleagues Bennett Simon and Donald Gerard, who read and criticized portions of the manuscript. Donald Gerard and Helmut Thomä assisted me with the translation of Freud's term *Nachträglichkeit,* which is central to the thesis that I develop in this book.

Finally, I wish to thank my wife, Penelope, for her editorial assistance and for providing me with the necessary environment.

Contents

Time present and time past
Are both perhaps present in time future,
And time future contained in time past.

—T. S. Eliot, *Burnt Norton*

Introduction

Of all the many aspects of psychoanalysis, Freud paid the least attention to the theory of treatment. His own theory of treatment can be inferred from his papers on technique, all of which were published between 1911 and 1915. Unlike his thinking about metapsychology, which evolved under the influence of clinical observation, Freud's theory of treatment, incomplete as it was, remained relatively static.

We now view the analytic setting and the analytic relationship as a major element in the curative process, yet Freud believed that the psychoanalytic relationship was not part of psychoanalytic technique. It is ironic that the psychoanalytic setting, Freud's most original contribution to the technique of psychoanalysis, is something that he took for granted and did not investigate further. Such a relationship, Freud thought, was no different from that encountered in other healing relationships such as those that exist between all doctors and their patients. He made only a brief and passing reference to this nonspecific therapeutic relationship, which he called the *unobjectionable positive transference*.

It must be said at the outset that we do not as yet possess a theory that explains how psychoanalysis works. When I was a student, such a theory of psychoanalytic treatment might have been viewed as superfluous, as if the therapeutic action of psychoanalysis hardly warranted an explanation. For it was an unquestioned assumption that psychoanalysis achieves its curative effect through the development and resolution of the "transference neurosis." Today we know that there is an entire class of neuroses, the so-called narcissistic disorders, in which the experience of the transference is quite different from that of the "classical" case in that a transference neurosis is either entirely absent or present in only a vestigial form. These observations have forced us to reconsider what the term *transference* itself signifies and have led many to believe that the concept of the transference neurosis is obsolete. Whatever the concept of transference signifies, if psychoanalysis cures by means of the transference, there is a further question: how does the "resolution" of the transference lead to therapeutic change?

My curiosity about this problem was aroused when I observed that for a certain group of psychoanalytic patients, significant therapeutic gains occurred in spite of the fact that they were relatively cut off emotionally both from me and from their own inner life. When patients are withdrawn there is little opportunity to make interpretations at the point of emotional urgency, which Strachey suggested was the explanation for the therapeutic action of psychoanalysis. It appeared as if nothing very much was happening in the treatment, yet for many patients a curative process was mobilized. I suggested that the therapeutic benefit might be explained by the fact that these patients were experiencing the analytic setup, which includes the analytic relationship, as a "holding environment," in Winnicott's use of the term. These observations have persuaded me that it is the psychoanalytic setting itself that is the foundation upon which everything else rests.

If Freud did not bequeath to us a comprehensive theory, he did however provide the elemental concepts of *transference, resistance,* and *interpretation* which any contemporary theory of psychoanalytic treatment must consider. Furthermore, Freud did conceive of an idea that has the potential to transform those familiar therapeutic elements into such a comprehensive theory. I am referring to the concept of *Nachträglichkeit,* a term that Strachey translated as "deferred action." Because Strachey's translation might be confused with the idea of abreaction, which is not at all what Freud intended, I have retained the German term rather than using Strachey's translation. What Freud intended to convey by means of the term *Nachträglichkeit* is that memory is retranscribed as a result of subsequent experience. This concept opens up a psychology of "subsequentiality," a psychology of cyclic rather than linear time. Transference obviously shares in this quality of subsequentiality (*nachträglich*), and if this idea is taken seriously we will have to revise our thinking regarding the linearity of psychic development. The application of *Nachträglichkeit* to the theory of therapeutic action will be examined in Chapters 1 and 4.

As a piece of intellectual history, the concept of *Nachträglichkeit* has had an interesting fate. This concept first appears in a letter (December 6, 1896) from Freud to Fliess and is explicitly referred to in the paper "Further Remarks on the Neuro-psychoses of Defense." It then became part of Freud's intellectual equipment; for example, the concept of *Nachträglichkeit* is essential to Freud's interpretation of the case of the Wolf Man. In that case history Freud describes a series of recontextualizations: the primal scene is witnessed at age one and a half; that memory is subject to *Nachträglichkeit* at age four and again during the patient's psychoanalysis with Freud as a young adult, which he initiated at age twenty-four. But in Freud's later work the concept seldom appears. I suspect that the idea of cyclic time was inconsistent with Freud's attachment to the theory of the death instinct, where time is treated in a more deterministic, linear fashion.

The concept of *Nachträglichkeit* is virtually unknown among American psychoanalysts. This may be due in part to Strachey's faulty translation; but this idea is also inconsistent with the belief in an orderly hierarchical psychic development such as that envisioned by ego psychologists. *Nachträglichkeit* is much better known among European analysts, perhaps as a result of the influence of Lacan, who fully recognized its importance.

Freud's deep insight that memory is retranscribed in accordance with later experience has received confirmation from an unexpected quarter. Gerald Edelman, a Nobel Prize winner for his work in immunology, has turned his attention to the neurosciences and has proposed a revolutionary theory of memory based on recent advances in that field. In Edelman's theory, memory is not a record in the central nervous system that is isomorphic with past experience; instead, memory is conceived as a *recategorization* of experience. In Chapters 1 and 4 I discuss the connections between Freud's theory of *Nachträglichkeit* and Edelman's theory of memory.

I have found Edelman's theory to have immediate relevance for psychoanalysis, for the theory proposes that past experiences are not recorded in the brain in a fashion that is isomorphic with those events; rather, what is stored is the potential to activate *categories* of experience. This provides the means for a fresh interpretation of the biological function of repetition; it is now possible to modify Freud's antiquated repetition compulsion, derived from his theory of the death instinct, in a way that is consistent with the findings of modern neuroscience. I discuss this topic further in Chapter 4. Edelman's theory of memory also has immediate relevance to the problem of affect repetition within the transference and countertransference. As a bridging concept between Edelman's theory and psychoanalysis, I have introduced the term *affect categories*. This concept will also be discussed in Chapter 4.

In this book I have broadly interpreted *Nachträglichkeit* to mean that *the ego is a structure engaged in the processing and reorganizing of time*, so that our therapeutic technique can be thought of as something designed to maximize the recontextualization of the experience of time. In Chapter 5 I discuss the experience of time itself and the differences between cyclic and linear time.

It has long been recognized that psychotherapy mobilizes curative forces that are present in ordinary life. Freud, for example, recognized that transference was a form of love relationship. But in considering transference love and the love relationships that are part of ordinary life, Freud was confronted with the distinction between illusion and reality. He described transference love as something that was both real and unreal. The analytic relationship itself can also be viewed as fundamentally paradoxical: it has been described as a "real" relationship, something in the here and now, and yet it is also believed to be capable of recreating the earliest aspects of mother-child interactions.

I have found it clarifying to apply the theory of play and playing as proposed by Huizinga and Winnicott to the paradox of the psychoanalytic setting and the psychoanalytic relationship, as I discuss in Chapter 2. Both Huizinga and Winnicott view play and playing as paradigmatic of an aspect of culture. Play is contained within a frame that holds an illusory space that is separate from that of ordinary life. I have also found it clarifying to think of the difference between the psychoanalytic relationship and relationships found in ordinary life as the difference between two levels of reality. Within this frame there occur certain enactments that I prefer to call *symbolic actualizations;* I present this as an alternative to the explanation that the therapeutic action of psychoanalysis entails a regression. Regression is not very frequently invoked today as an explanation of therapeutic action, but the idea of regression within the transference, or regression to a state of childlike dependency, was central to theories of therapeutic action proposed several decades ago by such eminent psychoanalysts as Greenacre, Spitz, Gitelson, Balint, and Winnicott. Thus the concept of regression is important at least historically, and for this reason the intellectual history of the idea of regression will be traced in an appendix to Chapter 2.

In Chapter 3 I extend further the concept of levels of reality. In this effort I have been influenced by the novelist Italo Calvino, who examined the significance of levels of reality in literature and made the important observation that *each level of reality acts upon another level of reality and transforms it*. From this point of view I have found it useful to think of the psychoanalytic setting, the "frame" of the analysis, when functioning well, as a container of other levels of reality. Different forms of the transference can be thought of as different levels of reality. When these levels of reality are apperceived separately they can be contained within the frame, in which case we recognize the presence of a "therapeutic alliance." When such levels of reality become confused, transference interpretations are necessary to restore the frame of the analysis. I have substituted the term *iconic/ projective transference* for the more familiar term *transference neuroses*. The psychoanalytic setting is itself a form of transference that I have termed the *dependent/containing transference*.

There are complex effects, meanings, and functions that follow from the act of interpretation. This subject is examined in Chapter 6. Not only does the analyst, by means of interpreting, reestablish the frame of the psychoanalysis; the analyst also introduces his or her own *construction* of reality. This leads to the question: whose reality is interpreted, the analyst's or the analysand's? Is the content of the interpretation only the analyst's construction, as some have maintained, or does the content of the interpretation reflect the analyst's perception of the *patient's* mind?

There is an inherent conflict between the child's construction of reality and the construction of reality that is presented from without. A similar conflict is revived when the analyst makes interpretations, so that the subject of interpretation inevitably leads to the broader question: how does one learn from others? The Russian psychologist Vygotsky proposed (Bruner 1985, p. 24) that "the tutor or aiding peer serves the learner as a vicarious form of consciousness until such time as the learner is able to master his own action through his own consciousness and control" (see Chapter 6). In psychoanalysis, some individuals require the continued presence of the analyst in order to make use of the analyst's consciousness. We describe such conditions as a character deficit, which may make the analysis interminable.

The fundamental elements of psychoanalytic treatment as outlined by Freud are transference, interpretation, and resistance. From the standpoint of a theory of treatment, I have found the concept of resistance to be the least satisfactory. Although any theory of therapeutic action must consider those forces that are opposed to change, Freud's concept of resistance includes too much, encompassing the entire psychic apparatus. He lists five kinds of resistance—three emanating from the ego, the others from the id and superego. What I present instead, in Chapter 7, is an examination of resistance from the perspective of the schizoid defense of non-relatedness. The defense of non-relatedness serves multiple functions, one of which is a defense against the intrusion of the parent's construction of reality. For some individuals, when they were children, the acceptance of the parent's construction of reality may have been experienced as a threat to the continued existence of the self. Yet, paradoxically, this state of non-relatedness in the presence of the analyst can promote healing. What I have observed is similar to Winnicott's paradox: that the capacity to be alone requires the presence of another person. When this process is the dominant mode of relatedness, I have described it as a *sphere within a sphere*.

We know that each patient makes use of treatment in his or her own distinctive fashion. This could lead to a multiplicity of theoretical models. In Chapter 8 I adopt another strategy, describing the variable use that patients make of their treatment as a correlate of different modes of relatedness. In this, I have been influenced by Winnicott's idea that the use of an object is a developmental achievement. One can discern developmentally "higher" and "lower" levels of relatedness; these modes of relatedness may be characterologically fixed or fluid, dynamic, and rapidly changeable. One can contrast, for example, a patient's use of the therapist as a purely utilitarian (dehumanized) object with a mode of relatedness where there is a shared creativity based on the patient's capacity to merge playfully and yet remain separate. In this chapter I also reexamine the concept of the therapeutic alliance and suggest that it is, in part, dependent on the analysand's borrowing the analyst's acceptance of the paradox of the presence of multiple levels of reality within the therapeutic setting.

It is evident that paradox permeates the psychoanalytic process. In Chapter 9 I focus on the subject of paradox itself. Although the patient may accept the paradox of transference, paradox engenders insoluble therapeutic dilemmas. For example, gratification by means of the transference leads to the dilemma that gratification at one level of reality produces frustration at another level.

The psychology of the self can also be viewed as a phenomenon that is fundamentally paradoxical: the experience of the self is essentially a private experience, yet the self is defined by others. Some have argued that for this reason we may need to apply a different logic to the therapeutic dilemmas that result from the psychopathology of the self. In Chapter 9 I discuss a variety of such therapeutic dilemmas.

There are many competing theories of psychoanalytic treatment that are not easy to categorize. These competing theories reflect controversies regarding the etiology of the neuroses, which lead, understandably, to differences of opinion regarding the aims of treatment. For those who view the neuroses as primarily traumatic in origin, the aim of treatment is ameliorative—to provide the patient with a "new" object and a second chance. For those who view the etiology of the neuroses as primarily intrapsychic, such gratifying procedures are looked upon with great distrust. In Chapter 10 I perceive such controversies to be a continuation of the quarrel that occurred between Freud and Ferenczi in the early 1930s. If one fully accepts the consequences of Freud's idea of *Nachträglichkeit*, these controversies become moot. The polarity between "deficit" models of psychoanalytic treatment and "conflict" models can then be seen as a false polarity. If one fully accepts the concept of cyclic time, then those who emphasize the importance of the here and now in the therapeutic experience, as opposed to a repetition of the past, are also creating a false dichotomy. If a theory can in any way shift our attention away from questions that are by their very nature insoluble, and enable us to focus on those questions that have a solution, then the attempt at theory construction will have been worthwhile.

1

Freud's Theory of
Psychoanalytic Treatment

I do not intend to present here anything resembling a full account of
the development of Freud's theory of psychoanalytic treatment. Instead, I intend to focus on those specific elements in Freud's theory
that have relevance for the thesis that I shall develop in the succeeding
chapters. I shall argue for the centrality of the psychoanalytic setting,
a setting that functions as a facilitating environment in which multiple levels of transference realities are experienced. By means of the
juxtaposition of these levels of reality, memories and fantasies are
recontextualized in accordance with Freud's idea of *Nachträglichkeit*.

Freud paid scant attention to the psychoanalytic setting itself because it was something that he took for granted. He did however
make a passing reference to the psychoanalytic relationship, which he
called the *unobjectionable positive transference*. Lipton (1977) believed that for Freud the analytic relationship was not part of technique. This is shown in his treatment of the Rat Man, when Freud fed
his patient the famous herring. In inviting the Rat Man to partake in
the family meal, Freud was not departing from "classical" technique,
as subsequent generations of analysts have claimed, because the analytic relationship was, for Freud, something apart from technique.
Lipton makes the point that the essential difference between modern
technique and Freud's is that the definition of technique has been
expanded to include the analytic relationship. It is my contention that
the analytic relationship, the psychoanalytic setting, is essential to the
therapeutic process in that it functions as a container for multiple
levels of reality. From this point of view it is of interest that Freud's
feeding the Rat Man had no apparent deleterious effect upon the

treatment; from which I would conclude that in this instance at least, he, the patient, had no difficulty in moving from an extraordinary relation to an ordinary relationship and back. Or, to rephrase it in the language that I shall shortly be using, the Rat Man had no difficulty in moving from one level of reality to another.

In his letters to Fliess and in the paper "Further Remarks on the Neuro-psychoses of Defense" (1896), Freud introduced the idea of *Nachträglichkeit,* which is central to my thesis. As I explained in the Introduction, the term does not mean "deferred action," as Strachey misleadingly translated it, but rather that subsequent experience results in a *retranscription of memory*[1] or a *retrospective attribution* (Thomä 1989).[2] In this context Freud presents us with a theory of nonlinear, cyclic time.

The Shaman and Hypnosis

Psychological treatment has probably existed from the very beginning of culture itself. We believe that the professional healer, the shaman, wizard, or medicine man, was never an ordinary person but someone set apart from everyday life and invested with extraordinary status within the community as a result of his knowledge, learning, skill, and the arduous apprenticeship that preceded his investiture. The shaman is a particular type of medicine man whose powers are believed to be derived from his intercourse with envisioned spirits, which usually occurs during adolescence. This intercourse with spirits is not infrequently the result of a severe psychological breakdown, which then serves as a precondition for the role of shaman (Campbell 1983).

The patient placed his hopes not in the medications or curative techniques but in the *person* of the healer, so that the healer's personality was the principal agent of cure. Whether the treatment was directed against physical or psychological illness, the method of treatment, without discounting the value of primitive pharmacopoeias, was essentially psychological, for in primitive societies there is no Cartesian distinction between mind and body.

These early methods of psychological treatment not infrequently included altered states of consciousness in which the patient was put into a trancelike condition, not unlike the altered states of consciousness that accompany hypnosis. The aim of the treatment was the removal of the disease-producing agent. There is a famous account of

Boas's report of a Kwakiutl shaman cited by Ellenberger (1970, p. 10): "[The shaman] feels the patient's chest and wets his mouth; he then sucks the place where he has localized the sickness. After a while, he takes from his mouth something looking like a bloody worm, declaring that he has extracted the 'disease,' after which he sings his sacred song." Boas's narrator explained that in the curriculum of the four-year school for shamans, the students are taught to create the "bloody worm" by putting some eagle down in the corner of their mouth, which they then mix with blood by biting their tongue or rubbing their gums. Although the extraction of the "disease" is a trick or illusion, the cure depends on the patient's faith in the authenticity of the healer.

We can observe in this account certain familiar elements of psychological treatment. The attention of the patient is focused on the person of the therapist, who is endowed with special qualities that separate him from others in ordinary life. The therapeutic setup is designed to promote the intensification of illusions. There is a theory of pathogenesis in which the noxious agent is transferred from the body of the patient to the body of the therapist—a primitive transference. The idea of removing noxious products from the inside of the patient is not unlike the importance attributed to the removal of pathogenic ideas and fantasies.[3]

In this description of primitive healing the influence of the shaman is inseparable from those qualities attributed to him by the patient; that is to say, the cure depends upon transference. The term *transference* has many connotations: in the most concrete sense, transference means that which is displaced, that is, *transferred,* onto the person of the therapist. In the model of the shaman's treatment something is literally transferred (by means of an illusion) from patient to shaman: an illusion that some noxious element, something alien from within the patient's self, is transferred, exteriorized, and placed into the body of the therapist. In the process of transferring the noxious agent into the therapist, we might also infer that the patient experiences an illusionary sense of connection and perhaps merging with the shaman, which reinforces the sense of magical contiguity with the power of the numinous healer. The power of the shaman is not unlike the authority of the hypnotist, an authority that is explained by the term *suggestion,* although we still do not really know what that term signifies.

Freud's theory of psychoanalytic treatment was influenced by the fact that he practiced hypnotism for approximately seven years, from 1886 to 1893, before he became a psychoanalyst. Jones (1953) described him as championing the cause of hypnosis in that he translated Charcot's lectures into German as well as two volumes of Bernheim's treatise on suggestion and its therapeutic effects. Chertok and de Saussure (1979), in their review of the eighteenth- and nineteenth-century literature on hypnosis, indicate that Freud may have borrowed more from this literature on hypnosis than is generally recognized. Many fundamental ideas concerning psychoanalytic treatment were prefigured in these studies of hypnosis and what was earlier referred to as "animal magnetism." These eighteenth- and nineteenth-century hypnotists knew, for example, that the relation between the hypnotist and his subject was a form of love relationship. Further, they knew that this love relationship had erotic, dependent, and regressive characteristics, the last two qualities recreating aspects of a parent-child relationship in accordance with the hypnotic subject's credulous, submissive, and obedient attitude.[4] Chertok and de Saussure provide historical evidence that the idea of a therapeutic cure through transference love did not originate with Freud. For example, they quote from Binet in 1888: "The magnetized subject is like a passionate lover for whom there exists nothing else in the world but the loved one" (Chertok and de Saussure 1979, p. 136). That others before Freud had recognized that the relation between the hypnotist and his subject was a type of love does not in any sense depreciate Freud's contribution, however; for without Freud's creation of the *concept* of transference, these observations would have no meaning or significance.

The Case of Anna O. (Bertha Pappenheim)

Anna O., an extraordinary woman, a self-created ur-analysand, discovered a method of treatment which she then shared with her physician, Josef Breuer (Breuer and Freud 1893). She called this the "talking cure" or "chimney sweeping," and she is credited with discovering that catharsis can cure severe hysterical symptoms. However, this curative technique is by no means identical to free association, although it was its most immediate precursor. Anna O. discovered, under a state of auto-hypnosis, that if she recounted in detail the circumstances surrounding the onset of a symptom, that symptom would be relieved. For example, she told Breuer how her difficulty in swallowing water started after she had seen a dog drinking from her glass, and in the recounting she removed the symptom. In this fashion Breuer and his patient laboriously traced back to their origin each of her multiple, complex, and severely debilitating symptoms. They finally reached the root cause of her illness when they discovered that when Anna O. was nursing her father in his terminal illness, she was sitting at his bedside with her right arm over the back of a chair. She fell into a waking dream in which she saw a black snake coming toward her father as if to bite him. She tried to keep the snake from him, but her right arm, draped over the back of the chair, was in actuality deprived of its circulation and had consequently become semi-paralyzed. Coincidentally she uttered a prayer in English: during her illness she responded only to English and forgot her native German. She continued to have a hemiparesis of the right arm and suffered from hallucinations of black snakes. Following the narration of the origin of her symptoms to Breuer, all of those symptoms were relieved: the hemiparesis of the right arm, the terrifying hallucinations of black snakes, and her abandonment of her native language. Although Anna O. was not as completely cured as Breuer had supposed, the fact that even a partial cure had occurred is in itself quite remarkable considering the severity of her illness.

The symptoms just described are only a partial account of a vast museum of symptoms that developed in connection with her father's fatal illness, including a paralysis of three limbs with contractures and anesthesia, disturbances of speech, ocular disturbances, and a nervous cough. Anna O. also had a "double personality" with two distinct states of consciousness. In one of these states she was relatively normal, although melancholic and anxious, while in the other state she was "naughty" (abusive) and would hallucinate. These two personalities were sharply distinct, the main feature being that the sick personality lived 365 days earlier than the healthy one. Breuer described her as having the capacity to induce within herself an alternation between these two states of consciousness; or Breuer could induce a change of consciousness himself by confronting her with an object that was associated with the trauma of the previous year. For example, to switch from one state of consciousness to the other, Breuer had only to hold up an orange (oranges were the only food that she lived on during the first part of her illness). The sight of the orange would then induce her to leave the current year, 1882, and return to the previous year, 1881. The events of the previous year that she reenacted in this altered state of consciousness corresponded exactly to the actual events, as confirmed by a diary of her illness that her mother had maintained.

In contrast to the shaman's cure, Anna O.'s treatment was a collaborative effort; indeed, it was Anna who instructed Breuer on the technique of "chimney sweeping." But even though Anna O. discovered the method of cure, she could not heal herself without Breuer's protective presence. The cure was dependent upon a strong positive transference, what Freud would later describe as the *unobjectionable positive transference*. But there was something else in addition to the unobjectionable positive transference; there was, as is now well known, a highly eroticized transference with which Breuer was unable to cope. Breuer, quite understandably, omitted all reference to this erotic relationship that formed part of the treatment. This hiatus in the account of Anna O.'s treatment was repaired by Freud, who supplied the missing details in conversation with both Strachey and Jones. Strachey recounts, in a footnote (Breuer and Freud 1893, p. 40), that Freud told him that when the treatment apparently reached a successful end, the patient manifested an unmistakable sexual transference. It was this, Freud believed, that led Breuer to postpone publication of Anna's case history and ultimately led to Breuer's breaking off all further collaboration with Freud. Jones adds to this account that Anna was not only very intelligent but also extremely physically attractive, to the extent that she inflamed the heart of the psychiatrist in charge of the sanatorium to which she was sent (Jones 1953, pp. 224–225). Breuer became so engrossed in Anna O.'s case that his wife became intensely jealous of Anna. When Breuer recognized the source of his wife's jealousy, his reaction was intense. The final "untoward event" (mentioned in Freud's "Autobiographical Study") was described by Jones as follows: one evening Breuer found his patient in the throes of a hysterical childbirth (pseudocyesis), the termination of a phantom pregnancy induced by the putative father, Breuer. This so unnerved Breuer that, according to Jones, he fled the house in a cold sweat. The next day Breuer and his wife left Vienna for a second honeymoon in Venice.[5]

Anna O.'s treatment, while containing some of the elements present in a contemporary psychoanalysis, was not a psychoanalysis.[6] Yet we can identify certain elements, or the precursors of certain elements of the therapeutic process, that are present in contemporary psychoanalysis. Traumatic memories are relieved of their pathogenicity

when reexperienced within the protective environment of the therapeutic relationship. Although contemporary treatment does not make
use of an altered state of consciousness, a state that Breuer called the
hypnoid state, it achieves its result instead by means of the transference. But in both instances there is an *alteration in the experience of
time*. In the case of Anna O. the transference was not used, as in
contemporary psychoanalysis, as a means of contrasting past and
present objects; instead, the shift between past and present was accomplished by means of hypnosis (the self-hypnosis practiced by
Anna and the direct hypnosis induced by Breuer). Recall that Anna
created this experience for herself by entering into an altered state of
consciousness in which the events of the traumatic year 1881 were
relived with an uncanny accuracy. Anna's auto-hypnosis resulted in a
shift from present time to the previous year, a process analogous to
the contrast between present and past objects that patients experience
today through the transference and its interpretation. Breuer believed
that the curative process depended in some fashion upon this altered
state of consciousness. Freud, on the other hand, disagreed with
Breuer regarding the existence of the hypnoid state (Freud 1905,
p. 27), which he described as superfluous and misleading.[7]

The aim of Anna O.'s treatment shares something with the shaman's treatment in that in both instances an effort is made to expel
the noxious, disease-producing agent. Breuer called this pathological
process a "retention hysteria," hence the cathartic treatment. For
Breuer, the analogue of the "bloody worm" was the "etiological
significance of affective ideas, deprived of their normal reaction,
which operate permanently *like psychical foreign bodies*" (my emphasis; from Breuer's letter to August Forel, November 21, 1907,
cited in Cranefield 1958, p. 319).

From Hypnosis to Free Association

Freud's theory of psychoanalytic treatment has nearly been reduced, in the popular mind, to an aphorism: "where id was there
shall ego be" ("New Introductory Lectures," Freud 1933, p. 80). By
extending the domain of the ego over the instincts and over the superego, the power of truth and knowledge will subdue the forces of
irrationality and thus provide the individual with the possibility of
greater freedom of action. In short, psychoanalysis cures by means
of insight, by making the unconscious conscious. Insight protects the

individual from being passively "lived through" by forces that are inevitable, unknown, and uncontrollable. Such aphoristic renderings of Freud's theory of therapeutic action do not do justice to the complexity and subtlety to be found in the Freudian texts.

The introduction of the method of eliciting free associations by instructing the patient to adhere to the fundamental rule of free association was initially recognized by Freud to be an alternative to the altered state of consciousness induced by hypnosis ("Two Encyclopaedia Articles," Freud 1923, p. 238). Freud abandoned hypnosis and the method of catharsis because the success of this method was entirely dependent on the patient's (positive) relationship to the physician, and if that relation was disturbed, all the symptoms of the patient reappeared. For hypnosis did not deal with the forces of resistance, especially transference resistance. Freud's use of the method of free association was also supported by a strong belief in the "strict determination of mental events" (1923, p. 238). This new method, this "psycho-analysis," was, according to Freud, primarily an art of interpretation, which required as a counterpart the psychoanalyst's *evenly suspended attention*. The expectation was that the patient's uncontrolled network of associations would provide a path that would enable the analyst to make an interpretation. The analyst's interpretation would then lift the barrier of repression.

Nachträglichkeit: The Retranscription of Memory

When psychoanalysis was first employed in the cure of symptomatic hysteria, the content of that which was under repression was believed to be the memory of a childhood sexual seduction by a caretaking adult, that is, the memory of a sexual trauma. A widely held view is that what is lifted from repression by means of the psychoanalytic treatment is the memory of the initial traumatic event, which was subsequently reunited with the affect that had become dissociated and "converted" into a bodily symptom. However, Freud himself casts doubt upon this relatively simple and straightforward account. Freud's theory of *Nachträglichkeit* is a theory of memory that affirms the experience of human or cyclic time in contrast to time's linear arrow.

The first indication of this concept appears in the "Project for a Scientific Psychology" (1895, p. 356), where Freud states: "We invariably find that a memory is repressed which has only become a trauma by *deferred* [*sic*] action." In a letter to Fliess dated December 6, 1896, we find the following (Masson 1985, p. 207):

> As you know, I am working on the assumption that our psychic mechanism has come into being by a process of stratification: the material present in the form of memory traces being subjected from time to time to a *rearrangement* in accordance with fresh circumstances—to a *retranscription*. Thus what is essentially new about my theory is the thesis that memory is present not once but several times over, that it is laid down in various kinds of indications ... I should like to emphasize the fact that the successive registrations represent the psychic achievement of successive epochs of life. At the boundary between two such epochs a translation of the psychic material must take place. I explain the peculiarities of the psychoneuroses by supposing that this translation has not taken place in the case of some of the material, which has certain consequences.

As discussed earlier, I believe that Freud's reference to a *retranscription* more accurately captures the meaning of *nachträglich*.[8] Freud publicly introduced these ideas, which he had previously shared only with Fliess, in "The Neuro-psychoses of Defense" (1896, p. 164): "It is not the experiences themselves which act traumatically but their revival as a *memory* after the subject has entered sexual maturity." This theory of *Nachträglichkeit* is a recognition that psychic time is not the equivalent of objective, linear time; time is circular; once is not enough.[9] In "Sexuality in the Aetiology of the Neuroses" (1898, p. 281) Freud states (concerning sexual traumas) that

> they produce their effect only to a very slight degree at the time at which they occur; what is far more important is their *deferred* effect, which can only take place at a later period of growth. This deferred effect originates—as it can do in no other way—in the psychical traces which have been left behind by infantile sexual experiences. During the interval between the experiences of those impressions and their reproduction (or rather, the reinforcement of the libidinal impulses which proceed from them), not only the somatic sexual apparatus but the psychical apparatus as well has undergone important development: and thus it is that the influence of these earlier sexual experiences now leads to an abnormal psychical reaction, and psychopathological structures come into existence.

Memories are constantly remodeled, as Freud remarked, in a manner "analogous in every way to the process by which a nation constructs legends about its early history" (1909, p. 206). The meaning of the original trauma is reconstructed when the child discovers its own genital sexuality.[10] If we put aside the specific issue of sexual trauma, the principle that Freud proposed is: *the ego can constantly remodel memory in accordance with current and immediate experience.* This principle has obvious relevance to the transference neurosis, which Freud would later refer to as a new construction, a newly created and transformed neurosis (1917, p. 444):

> Thus the transference may be compared to the cambium layer in a tree between the wood and the bark, from which the new formation of tissue and the increase in the girth of the trunk derive. When the transference has risen to this significance, work upon the patient's memories retreats far into the background. Therefore it is not incorrect to say that we are no longer concerned with the patient's earlier illness but with a newly created and transformed neurosis which has taken the former's place.

Transference, then, unquestionably belongs to the class of phenomena described under the heading *Nachträglichkeit*. The current interest as to whether the transference is a repetition of the past or a newly formed creation thus misses the point of the complex cyclic relation between affective memories and fantasies that are evoked by current reality. Transference is fundamentally paradoxical because it is the experience of cyclic and not linear time. Much of the current debate concerning the veridical quality, that is, the historicity, of the transference also needs to be reexamined in the light of Freud's idea of *nachträglich*.

Freud was fully aware of the complex relation between memory and fantasy, as he illustrated in the case histories of the Rat Man and the Wolf Man. Not only are memories remodeled by current experience, but fantasy may be used to fill in gaps in the memory record. In the case of the Rat Man, Freud showed (1909, p. 208n.) how the *nuclear complex of the neurosis* (fantasies derived from the Oedipus complex) is uniform in its content, reflecting the fact that these fantasies are not necessarily molded by experience. It follows then that the recreation of the nuclear complex in the transference may not necessarily be a repetition of experience but a recreation of a fantasy. In the "Introductory Lectures," Freud was explicit in noting that it would be incorrect to conclude that the transference is a literal repetition. He cited the example that the presence of a strong father transference does not necessarily imply that the patient had suffered previously from a similar powerful unconscious attachment of libido to his father (1917, pp. 455–456): "His father-transference was merely the battlefield on which we gained control of his libido: the patient's libido was directed to it from other positions. A battlefield need not necessarily coincide with one of the enemy's key fortresses . . . Not until after the transference has once more been resolved can we reconstruct in our thoughts the distribution of libido which had prevailed during the illness."

Freud appears to be suggesting that *the ego is a structure engaged in the processing and reorganizing of time.* This deep insight, which is revealed both in the early papers on psychoanalysis and in the case histories, may have been overshadowed and in part vitiated by Freud's later attachment to the theory of the death instinct, in which time is treated in a more deterministic, linear fashion. It is perhaps for this reason that the importance of *Nachträglichkeit* has not been sufficiently recognized.[11]

Freud's idea of *Nachträglichkeit,* a retranscription of memory, has received confirmation recently from a theory of memory proposed by Gerald Edelman (1987) that promises to revolutionize the neurosciences.[12] Edelman challenges the belief that the central nervous system contains a record of memory traces that is isomorphic with the events as perceived (1987, p. 204): "Inasmuch as it is the *procedure* by which memory operates that determines the issue, and in view of the assertion that memory is a form of *re-categorization* based on global mappings, long-term synaptic changes do not necessarily correspond to long-term memory. Nonetheless, it must be shown how, on the average, a categorical memory with durations up to years can be constructed from less long lasting synaptic changes in the network." By *procedure,* Edelman is referring to the dynamic interchange between categorical memory and the perception of the environment. As I shall describe in further detail in Chapter 4, Edelman believes the organism's motor activity to be an integral part of the perceptual system. Thus Freud's concept of *Nachträglichkeit* receives a neurophysiological backing from Edelman (1987, p. 211): "This is an *active* process in which behavioral action provides a continual test of new environments as well as a means of rehearsal for older mappings."

Rosenfeld (1988, p. 193) comments on the overall implications of Edelman's theory as follows: "Each person according to [Edelman's theory] is unique; his or her perceptions are to some degree creations and his or her memories are part of an ongoing process of imagination. A mental life cannot be reduced to molecules. Human intelligence is not just knowing more, but reworking, recategorizing, and thus generalizing information in new and surprising ways."

The Paradox of Transference

Freud observed that the transference is both a reality and an illusion but apparently did not comment on the fact that he was describing a paradox and hence gave contradictory advice. In his paper on transference love (Freud 1915), he asks the question: is the patient's love for the analyst genuine or is it an illusion? His first response is that it is no different from love outside of the transference, since all forms of loving are based on infantile antecedents, and woe be it to the analyst who scorns his patient's love or tells his patient that her love is not real. But then Freud goes on to say that in addition to the need for the analyst not to reciprocate the patient's love, he must treat it as something *unreal* because it is a love that has no analogy in real life (1915, p. 166):

> It is, therefore, just as disastrous for the analysis if the patient's craving for love is gratified as if it is suppressed. The course the analyst must pursue is neither of these; *it is one for which there is no model in real life* [my emphasis]. He must take care not to steer away from the transference-love, or to repulse it . . . but he must just as resolutely withhold any response to it. He must keep firm hold of the transference-love, but treat it as something *unreal* [my emphasis], as a situation which has to be gone through in the treatment and traced back to its unconscious origins.

This paradoxical transference love, the analyst hopes, will serve only as a proxy and not as an end in itself. Freud said (1915, p. 169): "He [the analyst] must not stage the scene of a dog-race in which the prize was to be a garland of sausages but which some humorist spoilt by throwing a single sausage on the track. The result was, of course, that the dogs threw themselves upon it and forgot all about the race and about the garland that was luring them to victory in the far distance."

There is no doubt that transference can also be understood as a manifestation of the compulsion to repeat—to recreate actively the pain that was experienced passively, to provide a second chance. Freud believed that the action of repeating the past within the transference was an inferior form of remembering (1914, p. 151): "The greater the resistance, the more extensively will acting out (repetition) replace remembering." That transference is both a new creation and a repetition confronts us with a different though related paradox, which I will examine in greater detail in Chapters 4 and 5.

Overcoming Resistance

How are the forces of resistance overcome? Freud's answer was that the repressing powers (the forces of the anticathexis) could only be overcome through love, that is, through the love of the analyst taken in its broadest context (1907, p. 90):

> The process of cure is accomplished in a relapse into love, if we combine all the many components of the sexual instinct under the term "love"; and such a relapse is indispensable, for the symptoms on account of which the treatment has been undertaken are nothing other than precipitates of earlier struggles connected with repression or the return of the repressed, and *they can only be resolved and washed away by a fresh high tide of the same passions* [my emphasis].

> Further light may perhaps be thrown on the dynamics of the process of cure if I say that we get hold of the whole of the libido which has been withdrawn from the dominance of the ego by attracting a portion of it on to ourselves by means of the transference (1917, p. 455).

Another paradox: resistance is overcome by means of transference love, but then transference love is also a resistance. To express it as a formula, one might say that facets of character resistance are converted into transference resistance, which can then be interpreted, but the interpretation itself can elicit fresh resistance. Resistance is not limited to transference resistance, inasmuch as Freud used the concept of resistance in many different contexts: as resistance to remembering due to the anticathexis of repression; as resistance to the acceptance of an interpretation; as resistance to the curative process in general, which he attributed to unconscious guilt and the secondary gains of illness. In spite of the multiple contexts of the term *resistance*, it was possible for Freud to describe resistance to remembering, in quasi-neurological terms, as a reflection of a quantum of energy that needed to be expanded if an idea was to remain outside of consciousness (Freud 1915). I find Freud's use of the term *resistance* to be unsatisfactory in that it is too inclusive, and does not distinguish intrapsychic processes (anticathexis) from the interpersonal processes of transference resistance. This will be discussed further in Chapter 7.

The Analyst's Insight and the Analysand's Insight

Although Freud never wavered with regard to the importance he attributed to insight, he made an important distinction between the analyst's insight and that of the patient. The latter occurs in a biphasic sequence. The communication of the analyst's insight is one step ahead of the patient's insight, but Freud added that the patient's acceptance of the analyst's understanding is dependent upon a measure of "suggestion" (1917, p. 455):

> Thus our therapeutic work falls into two phases. In the first, all the libido is forced from the symptoms into the transference and concentrated there: in the second, the struggle is waged around this new object and the libido is liberated from it. The change which is decisive for a favorable outcome is the elimination of repression in the renewed conflict, so that the libido cannot withdraw once more from the ego by flight into the unconscious. This is made possible by the alteration of the ego which is accomplished under the influence of the doctor's suggestion.

Acceptance of an interpretation in itself does not indicate whether or not the patient has succumbed to suggestion or exercised independent judgment. Freud believed that it is only by means of a reliving in the transference that the analysand obtains the conviction of the truth of an interpretation. The following statement is from "A Case of Homosexuality in a Woman" (Freud 1920, p. 152):

> In the second phase the patient himself gets hold of the material put before him: he works on it, recollects what he can of the apparently repressed memories, and tries to repeat the rest as if he were in some way living it over again. In this way he can confirm, supplement, and correct the inferences made by the physician. It is only during this work that he experiences, through overcoming resistances, the inner change aimed at, and acquires for himself the conviction that makes him independent of the physician's authority.

Freud says in effect that love for the analyst, the analyst's authority, or the analyst's suggestions are not sufficient for the patient to accept independently the truth of an interpretation; the truth of the analyst's interpretation must be supplemented by *a reliving within the transference, a reliving that confirms the specific content of the interpretation.*

The reality of the analyst's interpretation must ultimately be replaced by the patient's reality.

This biphasic account of the analyst's knowledge vis-à-vis the patient's knowledge has broad implications that touch on issues beyond the confines of psychoanalytic treatment. How do we learn from experience? How do we learn from others? Taking in or assimilating knowledge from another invariably entails an incorporation of the other's vision of reality. The analyst's insight corresponds to one view of the world, and the patient's insight corresponds to another; for some patients the acceptance of the analyst's interpretations carries with it all of the difficulties that accompany the acceptances of another's perception of reality. This problem becomes most evident in those patients who, in their childhood, found it necessary for their psychic survival to dismiss their parents' judgments of "reality" because they were able to perceive that those judgments were significantly and dangerously wrong. Thus, the question of the analyst's insight or the analysand's insight evolves into the question: whose reality is it? This subject will be discussed in Chapters 6 and 7.

The Unobjectionable Positive Transference

Freud described the "unobjectionable positive transference" as follows (1912, p. 105):

> Transference to the doctor is suitable for resistance to the treatment only in so far as it is a negative transference or a positive transference of repressed erotic impulses. If we "remove" the transference by making it conscious, we are detaching only those two components of the emotional act from the person of the doctor; the other component, *which is admissible to consciousness and unobjectionable* [my emphasis], persists and is the vehicle of success in psychoanalysis exactly as it is in other methods of treatment.

Much has been made of this brief statement (see, for example, Gill 1982), for this is Freud's only direct reference to what has come to be known as the "real" object relationship that exists between the analyst and analysand. It must be acknowledged that this relational aspect, which has become so central in contemporary psychoanalysis, was viewed by Freud as not deserving of comment. In the following chapter it will be seen that I have subsumed the unobjectionable positive transference within the larger heading of the psychoanalytic setting.

2

Play, Illusion, and the Setting of Psychoanalysis

The foundation of psychoanalytic treatment, upon which everything else rests, is the psychoanalytic setting. Yet this setting is something that Freud took completely for granted, even though it may have been his greatest contribution to technique, a more original concept than the method of free association. It is a truism that psychopathology places certain phenomena in sharp relief, processes that otherwise move silently or go unnoticed. For the "well-chosen"— that is to say, the "classical"—case, the psychoanalytic setting, although of great significance, is a silent presence and may be taken for granted by both the analyst and the analysand. With the "sicker" patient, however, the psychoanalytic setting itself becomes the central focus of the treatment and cannot be taken for granted. I suspect, as did Winnicott (1954), that when Freud formulated his theory of psychoanalytic treatment he was thinking primarily of those patients for whom the psychoanalytic setting was not itself a focus of conflict. If his theory of treatment had been based upon his sicker patients, a consideration of the psychoanalytic setting could not have been omitted.

The central importance of the psychoanalytic setting has been noted by Rycroft (1985, p. 123), whose views I can fully confirm: "Psychoanalytic treatment is not so much a matter of making the unconscious conscious, or of widening and strengthening the ego, as of providing a setting in which healing can occur and connections with previously repressed, split-off and lost aspects of the self can be re-established. And the ability of the analyst to provide such a setting depends not only on his skill in making 'correct' interpretations but also on his capacity to maintain a sustained interest in, and relationship with, his patients."

The psychoanalytic or psychotherapeutic setting is a conventional arrangement regarding time and space that has been established by psychoanalysis and psychoanalytic psychotherapy.[1] This setting is equivalent to what Stone (1961, 1967) called the "psychoanalytic situation," which he defined as "the common and constant features of the analytic setting, procedure, and personal relationship in both conscious and unconscious meanings and function" (1961, p. 9). At first glance it may seem incongruous to conflate the recurrent aspects of the physical arrangement with the personal relationship with the analyst. But in the patient's mind the constant and recurrent aspects of the physical arrangement of the psychoanalytic setting are experienced as a quality of the relationship to the analyst. Winnicott (1954, p. 285) demonstrates this fusion between the physical setup and the affective relationship in his description of the prototypical psychoanalytic setting as used by Freud, a description that is still valid.

> At a stated time daily, five or six times a week, the analyst would be reliably there, on time, alive, breathing. For the limited period of time prearranged (about an hour) the analyst would keep awake and become preoccupied with the patient. The analyst expressed love by the positive interest taken, and hate in the strict start and finish and in the matter of fees. Love and hate were honestly expressed, that is to say not denied by the analyst. The aim of the analysis would be to get in touch with the process of the patient, to understand the material presented, to communicate this understanding in words. Resistance implied suffering and could be allayed by interpretation. The analyst's method was one of objective observation. This work was to be done in a room, not a passage, a room that was quiet and not liable to sudden unpredictable sounds, yet not dead quiet and not free from ordinary house noises. The analyst (as is well known) keeps moral judgment out of the relationship, has no wish to intrude with details of the analyst's personal life and ideas. In the analytic situation the analyst is much more reliable than people are in ordinary life; on the whole punctual, free from temper tantrums, free from compulsive falling in love, etc. There is a very clear distinction in the analysis between fact and fantasy, so that the analyst is not hurt by an aggressive dream. An absence of the talion reaction can be counted on. The analyst survives.

The Reality of the Psychoanalytic Setting and
the Paradox of Transference

Because the psychoanalytic setting includes what the analyst does, it has been described as something "actual" or "real." Placing these terms in quotations indicates that there is some uncertainty as to their meaning. What do we really mean by "real"? Do we mean the psychoanalytic setting is "real" and that transference is "unreal," a distortion of reality? Such a line of reasoning would not carry us very far, for we would be soon faced with the problem: are there gradations in the degree of "realness"? It can be seen that this line of thought soon becomes absurd. And who is to decide, the analyst or the analysand, whether there is a distortion of reality? There is no absolute reality to which distortions can be compared.

There is another way of approaching the question of the reality of the psychoanalytic setting. Is the "real" bond that exists between analyst and analysand the same or different from that experienced in other relationships? How does one place this peculiar tie that is neither a friendship nor a love relationship? In what particular ways is it set apart from other relationships in life?

There are multiple levels of reality present in the therapeutic encounter, which in turn lead to multiple paradoxes.[2] The reader will recall the paradox implicit in Freud's account of the transference neurosis: that it was both something new, a creation of the treatment situation, yet also a repetition of the past. The same paradox is evident in descriptions of the psychoanalytic setting, which is also something that is actual in the sense that it is here in present time even though the object tie to the analyst can symbolically actualize aspects of the earliest stages of a mother-child relationship.

Transference has further paradoxical qualities in that it is both something unique, a nonrepeatable "happening," yet also a process that is repetitious. As the product of the total interaction (both conscious and unconscious) that occurs between the two individual participants, transference is unique. Yet it is also assumed that the form and content of the transference, or its absence, reflects character or structural psychopathology, and for this reason it is a repeatable configuration and can be used as a nosological marker. How can it be both a repeatable configuration and a unique happening? No one doubts that the reality of the analyst's personality—temperament, age, health, gender, and so forth—contributes to the content of the transference. In addition, the analyst's theoretical assumptions will influence which among the multitude of the analysand's responses will be selected or chosen to be avoided. All of this will accordingly mold the transference in one direction or another.

But it can be equally maintained that the form and content of the transference, or its absence, is a repeatable configuration irrespective of the unique interaction of the two participants. Naturalistic observations of the transference have long been an operational method of establishing nosological entities. Freud used the capacity or incapacity to form a transference as a means of separating the transference neuroses from what he then called the "narcissistic neuroses." This term is now obsolete, since Freud was referring to schizophrenia; he mistakenly believed that the schizophrenic withdrew to a state of a "primitive objectless condition of narcissism" and was incapable of forming a transference (1915, p. 197). Although Freud was mistaken, there is today widespread agreement that transference can be used to differentiate character and structural psychopathology. Thus we are left with the paradox: *transference can be hypostatized both as a repeatable configuration and as something that is newly created by the therapeutic encounter.*

Playing as a Differentiated Level of Reality

Freud assumed that the forces that produce change in psychoanalysis cannot be completely different from those forces that lead to psychological changes outside of treatment. Thus, the curative power of the transference can be seen as an extension of the curative power of love. From this point of view, the psychotherapeutic setting may be thought of as a means of concentrating those curative forces that are present in ordinary life. Another such curative force present in ordinary life is playing.

The great Dutch historian Huizinga has demonstrated that play is not something opposed to seriousness but rather that it is a fundamental aspect of culture. Huizinga viewed play or playing as a form of action contained within a separate reality, a reality set off and demarcated from that of ordinary life. Huizinga introduced his discussion with the following illustration (1950, p. 8): "A father found his four year old son sitting at the front of a row of chairs, playing 'trains.' When he kissed his son the boy said: 'Don't kiss the engine

Daddy, or the carriages won't think it's real.'"[3] Play, as Huizinga observed, has a fragile, ephemeral quality, a quality of illusion that is easily disrupted. It must be kept within its own frame, a frame that proclaims that playing occurs within a level of reality apart from that of ordinary life. This separation from ordinary life can be established in a variety of ways: playing takes place in a certain space and has certain limitations regarding the duration of time, as in games that are "played out" within a certain limit of time. Yet playing may have its own quality of timelessness. Playing is also separated from ordinary life by the "rules of the game": all play has its rules that pertain to the temporary world in which playing takes place. Rules are in effect a means of containing a space in which illusions can flourish. The connection between playing and illusion has long been recognized and, as many have noted, is revealed by the etymology of the word *illusion,* which can be traced to *inlusio, illudere,* or *inludere,* which means literally "in play."

Play is fundamentally paradoxical in that the essence of play is its freedom and spontaneity, but it is a freedom that must occur within certain constraints; all play is a voluntary activity, yet play is circumscribed and restrained by the "rules of the game" and the restraints of time and place. Play illustrates the profound truth that *freedom exists by means of restraints.* Playing transports the participants into another world, another reality, so that the concept of play includes much that is serious: "our ideas of ritual, magic, liturgy, sacrament and mystery would fall within the play-concept" (Huizinga 1950, p. 18). The anthropologist Leach echoed Huizinga when he noted that the bishop who dons his miter in the cathedral is not quite the same person as the one seen in a restaurant the following day (Leach 1986). Religion, which separates the sacred and profane by means of ritual and liturgy, can also be thought of as a form of playing. The psychoanalytic situation is also in this sense a form of playing in that it separates the participants from ordinary life. The problem, for both participants, is one of how to move from an ordinary relationship to an extraordinary relationship and back again.

I do not know if Winnicott was acquainted with Huizinga's work, but their views are remarkably similar. For Winnicott, playing also transcended the distinction between the serious and the nonserious, and he believed, as did Huizinga, that playing included cultural experiences: "I am assuming that cultural experiences are in direct continuity with play, the play of those who have not yet heard of games"

(1971, p. 100). As did Huizinga, Winnicott perceived that playing is at bottom paradoxical in that the freedom to play exists only within the constraints of a "set" situation. Winnicott (1958) observed infants at play, specifically in the spatula game where the infant's responses were observed within a controlled or set situation. The description is that of a normal baby, and variations from this norm are thought to be diagnostic. The child is on its mother's knee, and there is a shiny spatula on the table, for which the baby reaches. Winnicott does not give any active reassurance or initiate the first move, which is up to the baby. Later Winnicott would refer to the psychoanalytic setup as an analogy to the set situation of the spatula game. Of course, play in infancy does not consist of the set situation of a game. Play is spontaneous, but the capacity to play requires trust and confidence in the safety of the environment, which is provided by a maternal protective presence. I think of the mother's protective presence as a restraining boundary.

Winnicott's special contribution to the theory of play is his idea of *potential space*. He assumed, as did Huizinga, that the place where playing takes place is an area of illusion, a reality different from that of ordinary life. But what interested him most was the edges or margins between external reality and the internal realities in the minds of those who are playing. This theory of potential space is derived from Winnicott's concept of the transitional object, taken not in its literal sense as a protective or soothing object, but as a paradox in that an object can exist in the real world yet is the creation of the subject. Winnicott will often repeat ideas such as the following (1958, p. 239): "On the transitional object it can be said that it is a matter of agreement between us and the baby that we will never ask the question 'Did you conceive of this or was it presented to you from without?' The important point is that no decision on this point is expected. The question is not to be formulated."

This potential space represents the subject's transformation of external reality, creating something that belongs to neither "subjective" nor "objective" reality.[4] Within the potential space of the psychoanalytic setting there is the "objective" analyst as well as the subjectively created analyst; in a treatment that is functioning well, we do not ask the question whether the transference was subjectively created or whether it was presented from without. This potential space between subject and object, between analyst and analysand, where playing takes place, is a shared reality and we do not ask:

"whose reality is it?" An analysis functions well when one does not quite know whether it is the patient or the analyst who has made the interpretation. This potential space, this shared reality, is a playful or illusionary intermingling of the inner world of the two participants. As Winnicott said (1971, p. 38): "Psychotherapy takes place in the overlap of two areas of playing, that of the patient and that of the therapist. Psychotherapy has to do with two people playing together. The corollary of this is that where playing is not possible then the work done by the therapist is directed towards bringing the patient from a state of not being able to play into a state of being able to play."

For Winnicott, the aim of treatment is to provide a setting in which the patient is able to be maximally creative. Winnicott believed that the child's creativity could be impaired by mothers who did not accept the child's constructed view of reality. Resistance to the acceptance of the analyst's interpretations can thus be seen in fresh perspective: interpretations will be resisted not only because they confront the analysand with that which was painful or under repression, but they will be resisted because the interpretation is experienced as an intrusion of the *analyst's* world view, the analyst's construction of reality. For some patients, recognition of the analyst's creativity is experienced as a negation of their own creativity. Winnicott made the following observation (1971, p. 57): "My description amounts to a plea to every therapist to allow for the patient's capacity to play, that is to be creative in the analytic work. The patient's creativity can be only too easily stolen by a therapist who knows too much."

The reader will note that I have been using the term *reality* in two different contexts: one as a reference to *levels* of reality, such as the contrast between the psychoanalytic setting and ordinary life, and the other as a reference to a *constructed* reality. Huizinga and Winnicott understood that playing is a *shared* construction of reality, which takes place within a level of reality that is different from that of ordinary life. Winnicott's potential space is also a level of reality different from that of ordinary life that potentiates the intermingling of the constructed realities of the two participants.

There is good reason to believe that all cognition is a personal, idiosyncratic construction of reality (Piaget 1954). Piaget demonstrated that the child's cognitive development is a construction of reality which consists of a dialectic process of *assimilation* and *accommodation*. The former term refers to the "taking in" of the world in accordance with the child's internal schemata, while the latter term refers to the child's accommodation to external reality. There is no such thing as pure assimilation or pure accommodation. Transference also consists of imposing one's schemata upon external reality and yet accommodating to aspects of that reality (Wachtel 1980). Regarding the transference, one can say that there is no such thing as pure projection (construction), and there is no such thing as an unmediated response to external "reality" without reference to the internal world.

The Psychoanalytic Setting as a Frame

Marion Milner (1955, p. 86) was, to the best of my knowledge, the first to describe the psychoanalytic setting as a "frame" that functions like the frame of a painting, enclosing a separate reality. Some years later Bleger (1966), an Argentinean analyst, described the frame of the analysis as a "non-process" in the sense that it is made up of constants within whose bounds the process of analysis takes place— a description again consistent with Huizinga's theory of playing. Bleger's concept of the tacit constants of psychoanalysis can also be described as the "rules of the game"; these include the physical regularities of the therapeutic setup, discussed earlier, which are conflated with the object relationship with the analyst. Despite the spontaneity and unpredictability of the affective relationship between analyst and analysand, there are also certain affective constants that are institutionalized as part of technique and contribute to the frame or the rules of the game.[5]

Gregory Bateson (1972) pondered the implications of his observations of animals at play. He observed animals in a zoo engaged in mock fighting and reasoned that some sort of communication or set of signals must exist that would tell the participants: "this is only play"; "this is not ordinary life." For Bateson's animals at mock combat he presumed that there was some affective metacommunication that signaled: "this is only play," and he suggested that in the transference there is a similar metacommunication (1972, p. 191): "Just as the pseudocombat of play is not real combat, so also the pseudolove and pseudohate of therapy are not real love and hate. The "transfer" is discriminated from real love and hate by signals invoking the *psychological frame* [my emphasis]; and indeed it is this frame which permits the transfer to reach its full intensity and to be discussed between patient and therapist."

Bateson predicted that in some forms of psychopathology the individual may lack the capacity to accept the paradox of the concurrent existence of that which is within the frame and that which is outside. One can easily confirm his prediction in certain borderline patients and those with severe narcissistic character disorders, who cannot easily shift between the multiple realities of the transference, the therapeutic setting, and the (objective) characteristics of the therapist. In some instances these patients attempt to master this difficulty by engaging in provocative behavior that will eventually cause the therapist to retaliate or lose his temper, thus in a sense falling out of the frame. It is as if they need to obtain practice in shifting from one level of reality to another—a form of training to apperceive the presence of multiple realities. (This process will be discussed further in Chapter 4.) Some patients never permit themselves (or lack the capacity) to experience the illusion of transference, so that the therapist remains for them someone who is one-dimensional, literal, and concrete. Others accept only the relationship within the frame and cannot confront their perceptions of the analyst's reality. It can be said that these patients have great difficulty in accomplishing the act of moving from an ordinary situation to an extraordinary situation and back again; that is, they have great difficulty in accepting the paradox of the coexistence of separate realities. (The Rat Man, in contrast, had no such difficulty in shifting from the reality of an analysand to that of a person in ordinary life.) For many patients the entry into the consulting room or the space between the door and the couch becomes an intermediate area that belongs neither to ordinary life nor to the psychoanalytic setting, and it is here that the difficult transition between an ordinary and an extraordinary relation takes place.

The Affective Asymmetry of the Psychoanalytic Setting

I noted earlier that the freedom to play, paradoxically, requires certain constraints, certain rules of the game. Superimposed upon the physical setup—the patient reclining, the analyst sitting—is an affective asymmetry which contributes to the rules of the game and is also symbolically elaborated into transference manifestations that have been called dependent or "regressive." The affective constraints of the analyst are considered as part of technique; this includes the analyst's non-retaliation and the asymmetric mode of communication in which the analysand is asked to say everything while the analyst reserves the right of saying only what is judged to be in the best interest of the treatment. The therapeutic setup is designed to create an *asymmetry of need, desire, and communication.*

It is a truism that all human relations, as well as the relationships that exist between us and our domestic animals (Hearne 1986),[6] are established through the medium of affective communication. The analytic relationship is designed to be a communicative relationship; but it is unlike any other relationship in ordinary life.

Contemporary communication theory recognizes not only that the sender communicates (ostensive) information, but that there is in addition a simultaneous metacommunication, a message concerning the *relationship* between the communicants (Watzlawick, Bavelas, and Jackson 1967; Ruesch and Bateson 1951). We know that information concerning the relationship is communicated by means of the tone of voice, speech cadences, bodily movements, and so forth. The analyst responds to the affective charge of the spoken words and can observe that the communication of authentic affects is object-seeking (Modell 1984a); it is a communication of need. Conversely, the absence of authentic affects, words emptied of feeling, is a communication of the absence of need, of self-sufficiency. These metacommunications inform about the state of relatedness, the state of desire, that exists between patient and therapist. It is a further premise of communication theory that the absence of communication is a communication; this is expressed as the "impossibility of non-communicating." A state of non-relatedness, a state of withdrawal, may paradoxically coexist with an intense dependent relationship that remains unacknowledged. But the communication of non-relatedness may induce a corresponding non-relatedness in the analyst, which may lead the therapist to mistakenly minimize the extent of the patient's dependency.

What of the analyst's desires concerning the analysand? Most analysts desire to be useful and desire the furtherance and success of the analysis. But they also know that an over-zealous wish to cure is experienced as an intrusion of the analyst's agenda and inevitably becomes a focus of resistance. The analyst's needs and desires concerning the analysand also reflect the paradox of the simultaneous presence of at least two levels of reality—that of ordinary life and that contained within the analytic setting. To the extent that the patient is experienced by the analyst as someone in ordinary life, the analyst may wish the patient to be a source of narcissistic gratification or an object of sexual desire, or may experience the patient as a competitive rival, a source of envy, and so forth. In short, the analyst may experience the entire range of attitudes and affective responses that is present in ordinary life. But the analyst also functions within the frame of the psychoanalytic setting, a level of reality separate from that of ordinary life. Thus the analyst does not function as a person in ordinary life, who intrudes by taking action, who communicates desire, who retaliates; and these affective constraints contribute to the frame of the therapeutic setting. The analyst functions primarily in the best interest of the patient; what the analyst experiences, unlike the analysand, is communicated only to the extent that it serves the interests of the treatment. The analysand is expected to answer the analyst's questions, but the analyst may elect to remain silent in response to the patient's questions. There is an evident element of power and control here, as many have noted,[7] but in addition to that, this asymmetry will be experienced by the analysand as a form of symbolic action that reinforces the patient's dependency. This asymmetry of communication is analogous to a parent-child relationship in which parents tell children only what they judge to be in *their* best interest. But the children also learn that what is considered to be in their best interest reflects the parent's construction of reality.

Psychoanalytic technique is designed to facilitate the communication of the *analysand's* attitudes and desires toward the analyst, who, unlike a friend or lover, is expected not to retaliate, that is, not to act on the experience of an equivalent desire. Bion said that the analyst should approach each analytic hour without memory or desire. Apart from the fact that this injunction is impossible to fulfill, this Zen-like prescription contains an element of truth.

Neutrality as a Constraint

The technical injunction under which these potentially intrusive desires of the analyst are restrained comes under the heading of the analyst's *neutrality*. This term has at least two major connotations: one is implied in the term *indifferenz* used by Freud, which Strachey translated as neutrality (see Hoffer 1985 for a discussion of Strachey's translation of this term). This is consistent with the "scientific," objective distancing that Freud described as analogous to the surgeon's objectivity. The other connotation of neutrality is the absence of intrusiveness; that is, restraining the enormous potentiality of the analyst's influence over the analysand. This influence extends not only to the well-known problem of the analyst's introducing his own values and beliefs, but also to the analyst's use of power (Poland 1984). Neutrality in this sense protects the patient from the analyst's "eccentric intrusions." Neutrality was traditionally thought to preserve the "purity" of the transference, to minimize the impact of the analyst's personality; but we know now that to exclude the influence of the analyst's personality is impossible.

This distinction between the analyst as someone in ordinary life with ordinary emotional responses and the analyst functioning as an analyst (within the frame) has been described by Schafer (1983) as the analyst's having a *second self,* which he calls a fictive self. Calling the second self fictive implies that the analyst's analytic persona is not genuine or "real." Schafer draws the analogy between writer's empathy and compassion in her life as compared to the compassion, empathy, and depth of understanding displayed in her work. Mean-spirited writers may display considerable compassion in their work. Similarly, one knows of analysts who are very difficult human beings but function at their very best when they are sitting behind the couch. It is not that their analytic selves are fictive, not genuine, or less real; the analyst is not pretending. The analyst's second self simply represents a level of reality different from that of ordinary life. The analyst's persona as an analyst is not necessarily false, nor are the affects experienced within the frame of the analysis necessarily false. Bateson, from his observations of animals engaged in mock fighting in a zoo, drew the misleading conclusion that the affects of the transference are also mock affects, that the transference affects are only pseudolove or pseudohate. The point is not that such affects are false but that they occur in another context from that of ordinary life, within a different level of reality. (Transference affects can, of course, be false, but that is a separate issue).[8] An analogous situation occurs in dreaming. The affects that occur in dreaming are not in any sense less real than those affects occurring in a waking state; it would be hard to maintain that the anxiety or sexual excitation that occurs in dreaming is not real. The affects in a dream are real enough, but they occur within a different state of consciousness. The reality status of affects is an old problem, which Freud referred to in *The Interpretation of Dreams* (1900, p. 74). There he quotes an earlier authority, Stricker, as follows: "Dreams do not consist solely of illusions. If, for

.instance, one is afraid of robbers in a dream, the robbers, it is true, are imaginary—but the fear is real."[9]

But the fact that transference affects occur within a separate context may permit the patient to experience in this protected sanctuary, as Bateson suggests, that which they may not allow themselves to experience in ordinary life. The frame itself, even though it may be a silent presence, is experienced as a protective presence.[10] There is, in other words, an "as-if" quality to the analytic setting that permits some patients to express intense rage as well as intense sexual desire that they might not otherwise be able to express in ordinary life.

Dependency and Regression within the Frame

That there is, almost invariably, a dependent relationship between patients and their therapists is so obvious that it hardly warrants comment. But when we attempt to "place" this dependent relationship to the therapist, that is, to compare it with other dependent relationships, the matter is by no means self-evident or obvious. When one thinks of dependency one thinks of a parent-child relationship, and thus it has been customary to interpret this dependency as evidence that a "regression" has occurred. The concept of regression, although firmly entrenched in the literature, can be traced to certain antiquated ideas concerning biological evolution; thus the explanatory power of the idea of regression will not bear too much weight. Loewald (1981) says: "Words and concepts (such as regression and the rest) reveal themselves as flimsy or enigmatic or ambiguous if they are not merely used as shortcuts and as currency in the exchange of thoughts but are given weight and consideration in their own right."

One may sidestep the muddled thinking that is associated with the idea of regression by stating that this dependent relationship is only *analogous* to a mother-child or a parent-child relationship. But this raises the further problem: how is such an analogy established? Is the dependent relationship just a mimesis or a symbolic actualization, a kind of "play" contained within the separate reality of the therapeutic setting, or is there an actual temporal regression?

Many respected and authoritative analysts, such as Spitz, Gitelson, Greenacre, Balint, and Winnicott, in writing about the dependent relationship in psychoanalysis, retain a certain ambiguity regarding the question whether the description of the analytic relationship as a mother-child relationship should be taken only metaphorically or whether there is in fact a literal temporal regression. Spitz said (1956, p. 260):

> We have postulated that the analytic setting places the patient into an anaclitic relationship. I may be permitted to suggest a distinctive term for the role of the analyst in this setting. *Anaclitic* means leaning into: I recommend for the analyst's attitude the term *diatrophic*, which means supporting. *The diatrophic attitude has its origin in a developmental stage of the infant which emerges toward the end of the anaclitic relationship* [my emphasis]. The diatrophic attitude is a facsimile of the fantasies which belong to the stage in which the young child forms his secondary identifications with the parental figures.

Thus Spitz believed that the analyst's maternal attitude is evoked by the analysand's regression to an early infantile developmental stage. Greenacre expressed a similar idea (1954, p. 672):

> Even if the periods of repeated contact between two individuals do not comprise a major part of their time, still such an emotional bond develops and does so more quickly and more sensitively if the two persons are *alone* together: i.e., the more the spontaneous currents and emanations of feeling must be concentrated the one upon the other and not shared, divided, or reflected among members of a group. I have already indicated that I believe the *matrix of this is a veritable matrix; i.e., comes largely from the original mother-child quasi-union of the first months of life. This I consider the basic transference; or some part of primitive social instinct* [my emphasis].

Balint and Winnicott claimed that the analytic setting, when subject to regression, can recreate an early, indeed the earliest, mother-child relationship. Winnicott said (1958, p. 286): "The setting of an analysis reproduces the early and earliest mothering techniques. It invites regression by reason of its reliability." In "Birth Memories, Birth Trauma and Anxiety" Winnicott suggests that memories of birth trauma enter into the psychoanalytic experience when regression is a feature. Khan (Introduction to Winnicott 1975, p. xxii) quotes from a fragment of Winnicott's analysis of a forty-year-old female patient:

> A variety of intimacies were tried out, chiefly those that belonged to infant feeding and management. There were violent episodes. Eventually it came about that she and I were together with her head in my

hands. Without deliberate action on the part of either of us there developed a rocking rhythm. The rhythm was a rapid one, about 70 beats per minute (c.f. heartbeat), and I had to do some work to adapt to this rate. Nevertheless, there we were with *mutuality* expressed in terms of a slight but persistent rocking movement. We were *communicating* with each other without words. This was taking place at a level of development that did not require the patient to have maturity in advance of that which she found herself possessing in the regression to dependence of the phase of her analysis.[11]

The idea of regression was central to Winnicott's theory of the therapeutic action of psychoanalysis (1954, p. 281): "When we speak of regression in psychoanalysis we imply the existence of an ego organization and a threat of chaos. There is a great deal to study here in the way in which the individual stores up memories and ideas and potentialities. It is as if there is an expectation that favorable conditions may arise justifying regression and offering a new chance for forward development, that which was rendered impossible or difficult initially by environmental failure."

For Balint (1968) the concept of regression was also crucial. He attributed four functions to regression, regarding it (1) as a mechanism of defense; (2) as a factor in pathogenesis; (3) as a form of resistance; and (4) as an essential factor in psychoanalytic therapy. According to Balint, it is by means of regression that the "basic fault" is recreated and corrected within the treatment. The term *basic fault* is a geological metaphor suggesting that character formation is fundamentally flawed at the deepest levels, like a geological fault. Such a flaw is evidenced by a defensive withdrawal to the point where interpretations are experienced as dangerous intrusions. By means of regression the safety of an early mother-child relation is recreated within the transference, affording an opportunity to correct this basic fault. Winnicott proposed something similar in his conviction that the psychoanalytic setting functions as a holding environment and re-creates aspects of the earliest mother-child relationship.[12] For both Balint and Winnicott, the concept of regression was central to their theory of the therapeutic action of psychoanalysis. Although Winnicott fully appreciated the symbolic and metaphoric nature of regression, he believed that a literal regression to the earliest stage of life, including intrauterine experiences, was possible.[13]

Both Winnicott and Balint understood that the regression that becomes frozen into character formation is defensive but, more important, is also deeply adaptive. When regression reoccurs in the object relation with the analyst, it may provide the analysand with a second chance and a new beginning. Balint stated (1968, p. 136): "The analyst's role in certain periods of new beginning resembles in many respects that of the primary substances of objects. He must be there; he must be pliable to a very high degree; he must not offer much resistance; he certainly must be indestructible, and he must allow his patient to live with him in a sort of harmonious interpenetrating mix-up." (This "harmonious interpenetrating mix-up" is reminiscent of what Kohut [1977] would later describe as the "self-selfobject transference.") Balint said further (1968, pp. 70–71): "If any hitch or disharmony between subject and object occurs, the reaction to it will consist of loud and vehement symptoms suggesting processes either of a highly aggressive and destructive, or profoundly disintegrated nature . . . If we bear in mind that the ongoing harmonious relationship in this phase between subject and object or expanse is as important as the ongoing supply of air, we understand that loud, vehement, and aggressive symptoms appear when the harmony between the subject and its primary object or substance is disturbed."

Winnicott further described regression as a defensive withdrawal, a defensive "shield," a form of "self holding." If the psychoanalytic process succeeds in "holding" the analysand, it converts a "self holding" into a "holding" by the analyst (1958, p. 281): "It will be seen that I am considering the idea of regression within a highly organized ego defense mechanism, one which involves the existence of a false self . . . this false self gradually becomes a 'caretaker self,' and only after some years could the caretaker self become handed over to the analyst, and the self surrendered to the ego."

Symbolic Actualization

I have interpreted the therapeutic setting as a frame or enclosure within which actions take place that are experienced as separate from those of ordinary life. This description was influenced by the deep insight of Huizinga, who understood that play was such a separate reality and that playing included much more than games (1955, p. 10):

> . . . so the "consecrated spot" cannot be formally distinguished from the play ground. The arena, the card table, the magic circle, the temple, the stage, the screen, the tennis court, the court of justice,

etc., are all in form and function play-grounds, i.e. forbidden spots, isolated, hedged round, hallowed, within which special rules obtain. All are temporary worlds within the ordinary world, dedicated to the performance of an act apart.

Dependency that is evidence of the object relationship existing between analyst and analysand is no less real than dependency outside of the treatment, but it occurs within the frame of the psychoanalytic setting, a different level of reality. The reality status of the object tie to the analyst is paradoxical and consistent with Freud's old observation that the analysand's love for the analyst is both "real" and "unreal." The repeated and consistent actions of the analyst, analogous to rituals, provide the frame that separates analysis from ordinary life, but in addition these actions, experienced symbolically, intensify the analysand's dependency.

This is an alternative way of understanding regression. These preordained, repeated actions of the analyst include certain affective constraints that are part of the technique of psychoanalysis and contribute to what I have called the asymmetry of communication. The psychoanalytic setting is designed to maximize the analysand's communication to the analyst but not the reverse. The analyst's emotional position vis-à-vis the analysand follows this asymmetry of communication in that the analyst reveals to the analysand only what is judged to be in the best interest of the analysis. These "rules of the game" may be experienced by the patient as symbolic acts analogous to a parent-child relationship. There are further built-in constraints in the psychoanalytic and psychotherapeutic setting that symbolize or analogize a mother-child relationship. What the analyst actually does as part of ordinary "good" technique, without the introduction of active measures, creates the illusion of a protective parental relationship, a holding environment. This was the view of the therapeutic process which was originally proposed by Winnicott (1954), and which I have also elaborated (Modell 1976). These actions that may be experienced by the patient as symbolic equivalents of a parent-child relationship include the analyst's constancy and reliability, that he or she is always there listening; that the analyst is there primarily (but not exclusively) for the patient's needs; that the analyst's judgments are usually more benign and more objective than those of the patient; that not infrequently the analyst has a better grasp of the analysand's psychic reality than does the patient himself, and accordingly the analyst is able to clarify what is bewildering and frightening.[14] As a good mother does, the analyst contains the analysand's affective communications and tries not to retaliate.[15]

Within the frame of the psychoanalytic setting it is possible to recreate conflicts that have been observed in early childhood, such as the conflicts concerning merging and separation that are characteristic of the second and third year of life. The experience of merging and fusion not infrequently can be observed in the psychoanalysis of individuals who are not in any sense regressed in their lives outside of the analysis. This sense of being merged with the analyst can be observed in the opening phase (which may extend for several years) of the treatment of the narcissistic personality. At a certain point in the treatment the therapist frequently becomes aware that the patient expects to be understood without having to make the effort to communicate, something that is akin to the young child's expectation that his mother will understand him intuitively without the need for communication. For a considerable period of time the therapist may accept this expectation without comment; the patient in a sense is allowed to "live out" the experience of being merged with the analyst within the holding environment of the psychoanalytic setting. Sooner or later the analyst experiences, perhaps in response to the analysand's unconscious signals, a certain degree of impatience, not unlike the impatience of a mother of an older child who recognizes that the child is able but unwilling to take more responsibility for himself. The analyst at this point may tell the patient that he cannot be understood unless he is able to communicate. This intervention is experienced by the analysand as a confrontation with the fact that he and the analyst are indeed separate individuals. Although the patient may not welcome this intervention, it is one that may have been unconsciously manipulated by the patient to promote the process of individuation. I have described this type of interaction in *Psychoanalysis in a New Context* (Modell 1984a) as an illustration of what I call symbolic actualization: *the patient and analyst acting conjointly recapitulate early developmental phases.*

The term *symbolic actualization* owes something to a method of treating schizophrenia first described by the Swiss analyst Sechehaye (1951) as "symbolic realization." As a means of establishing contact with a severely autistic adolescent schizophrenic patient, Sechehaye introduced the use of symbolic "love gifts," such as ice to symbolize milk and a balloon to symbolize the breast. What is of interest is the observation that when Sechehaye attempted to use milk itself, the patient was unresponsive; it was essential that the patient utilize her *construction of reality*. Thus the efficacy of our symbolic acts depends upon a certain ambiguity that enlists the analysand's active participation in the creation of meaning.

These symbolic transformations are in themselves a form of transference. I have compared the psychoanalytic setting to a frame that encloses a separate reality, as does the frame of a painting. But this analogy begins to break down when one considers the fact that the psychoanalytic frame is not fixed and static but is itself subject to transformations, as I shall discuss further in the next chapter.

Appendix: Haeckel's Law and the Idea of Regression

The term *regression* itself derives from the verb "to go back," as in a journey, a return to the original point of departure, a reentry, a regress as opposed to a progress. It is a necessary term, when used simply as a description to denote the opposite of progress. But the term *regression* as used by Freud and subsequent generations of psychoanalysts is not simply a descriptive term but carries a considerable load of intellectual baggage, whose origins need to be examined. The concept of regression can be traced to certain ideas associated with nineteenth-century theories of evolution. These were ideas associated with evolutionary theorists other than Darwin, but they were nevertheless widely disseminated and had a profound influence on theories of psychology, child development, and penology as well as psychoanalysis (Gould 1977). Freud's thinking on this matter was most directly influenced by the work of the neurologist J. Hughlings Jackson and by Haeckel's now discredited biological law that ontogeny recapitulates phylogeny—an idea that Freud accepted uncritically, as did many of his contemporaries.

Jackson developed an evolutionary schema in which the nervous system was viewed as a developmental continuum from the lowest reflex center to the highest voluntary center, which culminates in the "organ of the mind" (quoted in S. W. Jackson 1969). This schema is that of a hierarchical system in which the less evolved, more primitive portions of the central nervous system are both succeeded and inhibited by the more evolved portions.[16] For example, if the cerebral cortex is damaged, its inhibiting effect upon spinal cord reflexes would be removed, leading to the emergence of archaic spinal reflexes. This ascending order was one from the simplest to the most complex, from the most automatic to the most voluntary, with the most recently evolved functions tending to be affected earlier while the older functions are affected later. Pathological formations can thus be viewed as atavistic and *regressive*. This manner of thinking has had a pervasive influence on psychoanalysis. In this schema of progress and regress within the central nervous system, Jackson was in turn influenced by Herbert Spencer's sweeping ideas that cycles of evolution are accompanied by cycles of dissolution (S. W. Jackson 1969). This idea that pathology, disease, or mental defect is a reversal of the order of evolutionary progress was a tacit assumption of nineteenth-century biology. Lombroso, for example, thought that criminal behavior was a return to an earlier developmental phase, since ontogeny recapitulates phylogeny, a perfectly normal child must pass through a savage phase as well (Gould 1977).

I do not intend to trace systematically the influence of these now antiquated biological ideas on Freud's thinking (for an extensive review of this topic see Sulloway 1979); it will suffice to recall that instincts as well as affects were thought by Freud to be precipitates of primeval traumatic experiences, the experiences not of individuals but of groups. These traumatic experiences were subject to Lamarckian inheritance[17] and transmitted to subsequent generations as a form of racial memory (Freud 1926, p. 93): "If we go further and enquire into the origin of that anxiety—and of affects in general—we shall be leaving the realm of pure psychology and entering the borderland of physiology. Affective states have become incorporated in the mind as precipitates of primeval traumatic experiences, and when a similar situation occurs they are revived like mnemic symbols."

The influence of Haeckel's law on Freud's thinking about the etiology of the neuroses can be seen most directly in the recently discovered missing metapsychological paper published as *A Phylogenetic Fantasy* (Freud 1987). In this paper, which Freud never published and did not intend to publish, Freud applied Haeckel's law in a stunning fashion. Freud saw neuroses as regressions, atavistic formations which contain a record of man's phylogenetic antecedents as well as the more recent history of mankind itself. The nosology of the neuroses, Freud believed, could be used as a record of the history of mankind, as if the neuroses were a window on the geological past (1987, p. 11):

It is still legitimate to assume that the neuroses must also bear witness to the history of the mental development of mankind . . . One thereby gets the impression that the developmental history of the libido recapitulates a much older piece of the [phylogenetic] development than that of the ego; the former perhaps recapitulates conditions of the phylum of vertebrates, whereas the latter is dependent on the history of the human race. Now there exists a series to which one can attach various far-reaching ideas . . . Ferenczi expressed the idea that the subsequent development of this primal human took place under the influence of the geological fate of the earth, and that the exigencies of the Ice Age in particular gave it the stimulus for the development of civilization . . . If we pursue Ferenczi's idea, the temptation is very great to recognize in the three dispositions to anxiety hysteria, conversion hysteria, and obsessional neurosis regressions to phases that the whole human race had to go through at some time from the beginning to the end of the Ice Age.

No one continues to believe that the history of mankind or the history of our remote ancestors, measured in geological time, is repeated in ontogenetic or developmental regressions. Yet Haeckel's law continues to have a subtle influence in psychoanalysis: it supports a belief in a literal temporal regression in the transference which otherwise would appear to be a nearly mystical expectation. Such a belief was implicit in the views expressed by Winnicott, Balint, Spitz, Greenacre, and others. Yet it must be admitted that we cannot do away with the assumption that, in one way or another, early developmental mother-child interactions are reproduced within the therapeutic setup. Since there are no facts that support a belief in a literal temporal regression, I have suggested an alternative explanation, that of symbolic actualization within a level of reality different from that of ordinary life.

3

Transference and
Levels of Reality

Throughout this book I will emphasize the fundamentally paradoxical nature of the psychoanalytic process, since paradox accompanies
the presence of multiple levels of reality. The paradoxical nature of
transference has contributed to its elusive quality and the lack of
clarity concerning the question of the patient's "real" relationship to
the analyst. This paradox that is transference has also contributed to
the confusion concerning the term *transference neurosis*. Experienced
analysts have expressed antithetical views concerning the therapeutic
action of the transference neurosis, some attributing therapeutic
change to a repetition of the past and others claiming that the neurosis represents a new creation. This confusion has resulted in the recommendation that the term be dropped altogether as an antiquated
concept (Cooper 1987). Because so much rests on the idea of multiple
levels of reality, it is necessary to examine in some detail what this
term signifies.

The experience of multiple levels of reality is part of our everyday
lives, but it is in literature that this concept becomes especially clear.
Italo Calvino (1986) made the important observation that *each level
of reality acts upon another level of reality and transforms it*. This
deep insight, congruent with Huizinga's theory of playing, can be
applied to the transference. As I described in the previous chapter, the
regularities of the therapeutic or analytic setup function as a frame
within which a separate reality is demarcated. But this separate reality
is also subject to transformation, so that the psychoanalytic setting
becomes transformed into another level of reality, the dependent/
containing transference.

In the previous chapter I described at least two levels of reality that are present in the consulting room: the analyst and analysand within the frame of the psychoanalytic setting, and the analyst and analysand as they are in ordinary life. This experience of different levels of reality not only is present in literature but is a narrative convention that is taken for granted. To provide a banal example: in the movies the narrative of the film is sometimes interrupted by a depiction of the protagonist's thoughts, fantasies, or daydreams—a representation of a different level of reality. This cinematic convention, a commonplace one that everyone accepts and understands, undoubtedly derives from the much older theatrical convention of the "aside" to the audience, where the audience understands that the actor is speaking the character's thoughts. The level of reality of the narrative action is temporarily interrupted, and the audience shares in the illusion that the other actors do not hear what is being said.

Multiple levels of reality can be even more clearly discerned in literature. Indeed, Calvino (1986, p. 101) defined literature as "an operation carried out in the written language and involving several levels of reality at the same time." As is true of life, there is no ultimate reality in literature; there are *"only levels."* Calvino teaches us that the interplay of levels of reality in a work of literature is extremely complex: the author inevitably interacts with his or her creation so that levels of reality involve not only the created work but also the author in interaction with that work. One must also consider the levels of reality in which the author chooses to speak. Calvino asks the question: who is the *I* who writes? *Is the I the author as "himself," or is the author an invention?* The *I* is always a projection of the author, but it may be a real part of himself or a mask. The same question has been asked about the analyst. Calvino provides this example (1986, p. 112): "Gustave Flaubert the author of the complete works of Gustave Flaubert projects outside of himself the Gustave Flaubert who is the author of "Madame Bovary" who in turn projects from himself the character of a middle-class married woman in Rouen, Emma Bovary, who in turn projects from herself that Emma Bovary whom she dreams of being." Analysts will have no trouble in recognizing here an analogy to the psychoanalytic process.

Calvino observes that these levels of reality may be kept separate or may melt, mingle, and be knit together. For example, in Shakespeare's *A Midsummer Night's Dream* the complications of the plot occur in three distinct but intersecting levels of reality: (1) the aristocratic characters at the court of Theseus and Hippolyta; (2) the super-natural characters, Titania, Oberon, and Puck; (3) the rustic comic characters, Bottom and his friends, who merge into the animal kingdom. Finally, there is a further level of reality in the play within the play—the story of Pyramus and Thisbe. Calvino contrasts *A Midsummer Night's Dream* with *Hamlet:* in the first instance the levels of reality are separate whereas in *Hamlet* they are fused. He describes *Hamlet* as a whirlpool that sucks in all the various levels of reality; it is from their irreconcilability that the drama comes into being. *Hamlet* also contains a play within a play; other levels include the realistic level of the narrative, Hamlet's awareness of his inner life, and Hamlet's "false" inner life, his feigned madness.

Two Forms of Transference: Dependent/Containing and Iconic/Projective

Calvino's deep insight, that each level of reality acts upon another level of reality and transforms it, illuminates what I have attempted to portray in the previous chapter. The tacit regularities of the psychoanalytic or psychotherapeutic setting create a frame that demarcates the therapeutic setting as a separate reality from that of everyday life. The analyst's actions as an analyst combined with the affective relationship to the patient that is regularized by technique are transformed by the patient's desires into another level of reality. The setting itself both contains another level of transference and is itself transformed.[1] There is a symbolic transformation of the reality contained within the frame. For example, there are commonly held illusions concerning the psychoanalytic setting, such as the belief that this setting functions as a protective alternative environment that stands between the patient and a dangerous world (Modell 1988a). The frame itself can be experienced as a transitional object. The content of this form of the transference is not idiosyncratic; it is nonspecific as compared to the nearly infinite variations of what has been traditionally referred to as the transference neurosis. The state of dependency regularly induces certain familiar, recurrent conflicts, such as the universal wish for merging union as opposed to the need to be separate and autonomous. In accordance with the patient's needs at a given moment, the analyst's actions may be experienced in different ways. The act of interpretation, for example, if it coincides with the patient's own thoughts, may be experienced as reinforcing a sense of merging union with the analyst; or, if the interpretation is perceived to be strange or outlandish, it will be experienced as a confrontation with separateness. In this fashion early developmental conflicts associated with the mother-child relationship are actualized. As discussed earlier, I do not think it is clarifying to characterize this process as a *regression;* instead I have described the recreation of early developmental conflicts as a process of *symbolic actualization.*

The transformation of the frame into another level of reality is perhaps most familiarly illustrated by the term *holding environment.* The experience of the analytic setting as a holding environment is not uncommonly elaborated further into the illusion that this setting functions as a protective alternative environment that stands between the patient and a dangerous world. This is truly a transformation into another level of reality that is not the "real" world, nor is it the world of imagination and pure fantasy. Perhaps this is what Lacan (1978) meant when he distinguished the real, the symbolic, and the imaginary.

Viewing the transference as the embodiment of many levels of reality helps to clarify the muddled and confusing issue of the reality status of transference and the reality status of the patient's relationship to the analyst or therapist. For decades there have been widespread disagreements concerning the reality status of the analytic relationship. For example, Anna Freud and Greenson have claimed that there is a relatively sharp separation between the analysand's attachment to the analyst, described as a "real" relationship, and the transference. Greenson (1970) found the "real" relationship difficult to define and admitted that all object relationships consist of different admixtures of the "real" and transference components. Nevertheless, he believed that the "real" object relationship was not transference. He defined transference as follows (Greenson and Wexler 1969, p. 28): "*Transference* is the experiencing of impulses, feelings, fantasies, attitudes, and defenses with respect to a person in the present which do not appropriately fit that person but are a repetition of responses originating in regard to significant persons of early childhood, unconsciously displaced on to persons in the present. The two outstanding characteristics of transference phenomena are (1) it is an indiscriminate, non-selective repetition of the past, and (2) *it ignores or distorts reality. It is inappropriate*" (my emphasis). Greenson assumes, then, that it is the analyst who is the ultimate judge of what is "real."[2] I believe that this controversy becomes irrelevant if one recognizes that the distinction is not between what is real and what is transference but between different *levels* of reality.

There is little disagreement, however, that the object relationship between patient and analyst is something quite different from what has been called the transference neurosis. Ever since Freud made his passing reference to the non-objectionable transference, there has been no difficulty in recognizing the existence of at least two major classes of transference. I have named the transference that is derived from the psychoanalytic setting, the frame of the analysis, the *dependent/containing transference*. This form of the transference differs fundamentally from what has been traditionally described as the transference neurosis. There is, I believe, widespread agreement on this distinction, which has been obscured by the variety of names applied to the dependent relationship: Stone (1967) called it the *basic transference;* Greenacre (1954) referred to the *primordial transference;* the transference/countertransference experience of this dependent relation was described by Spitz (1956) as the *anaclitic and diatrophic attitude;* and so forth.

I have added to the description of the dependent transference the term *containing,* in Bion's sense of transference as a container for the contained. Containing has multiple connotations. It can refer to the limits of the analytic setting—the rules of the game that apply to both participants; it also refers to the containing of affects. Containing also may mean accepting what is obnoxious to others or noxious to the self. The process of containing is not without its hazards: the container may not be adequate to what is contained, or the container may be pressured by the contents of the contained (Bion 1970). But in a broader sense, the illusionary space of the therapeutic setting, within which playing takes place, also *contains* other levels of reality, that is, other levels of transference; it gives rise to and contains another broad category of transference that is particularized and idiosyncratic. The psychoanalytic setting, when it functions as we would wish, creates and contains what I shall now call the *iconic/projective transference.*

To denote this particularity of the transference, in contrast to the nonspecific dependent/containing transference, I have introduced the term *iconic.*[3] This term connotes a visual portrait but may be used to express a representation, a similitude, that is not restricted to the visual sphere. Instead of pigment, the iconic transference uses affects as its raw material. I believe that the salient feature of what has been called the transference neurosis is the creation of another level of reality in which specific portraits of both internal and external actors emerge. The iconic transference may also create an interactive group portrait in that the analyst may be invested with the qualities of both subject and object. In this sense the iconic transference includes the concept of projective identification, the externalization of the record of affective interaction between self and object. (This process will be discussed further in Chapter 4.) The term *iconic* embraces both "imagoes" (a term used in the older literature to refer to whole, subjectively created persons—father, mother, and so on) and the internalized interactions with these objects that have been referred to as "internalized objects."

Piaget's distinction (1954) between assimilation and accommodation is relevant here—a differentiation that he considered to be biologically rooted and invariant. (For further discussion see Flavell 1963.) Accommodation is a response to what is *in* the environment. Piaget used the analogy of an organism ingesting food, where the organism must accommodate itself to the specific contours of what is being ingested. But once the food is ingested what is taken in is then adjusted, that is, assimilated by the organism, in that the organism imposes *its own schemata* on the foodstuff. Both accommodation and assimilation are always present, but not to the same extent. The dependent/containing transference can be described as predominantly accommodative, while the iconic/projective transference can be described as predominantly assimilative. The former is primarily a response to what is *in* the environment, whereas the latter is primarily an imposition of an internal schema upon what is presented from without.

The contrast between these two forms of transference can be schematically represented as follows:

Dependent/Containing Transference	Iconic/Projective Transference
Continually Present	Episodic or Absent
Symbolic actualization of developmental conflicts—Yes	Symbolic actualization of developmental conflicts—No
Recreation of specific idiosyncratic imagoes—No	Recreation of specific imagoes (including Oedipal)—Yes
Mutative interpretation—Enhances and strengthens	Mutative interpretation—Resolves or diminishes

Levels of Reality within a Transference Paradigm

Consider the following transference paradigm: A woman experienced her father as an absent presence during her puberty and early adolescence. When she was a little girl her father had taken delight in her. She remembered him as someone who was fun to be with, loving, and fully engaged with the family. During my patient's early adolescence, however, her father developed a serious depression and became emotionally unavailable; thus there was a very painful contrast between the father of the patient's early years and the depressed and withdrawn father of her adolescence. She never had the possibility of a satisfying adult relationship with her father because he died suddenly in her late adolescence from an unsuspected illness.

These facts serve as the background to a psychoanalytic session just prior to the start of my winter vacation, when this patient said: "You don't love me—you think that I am ugly." Later in the same hour she said more directly: "I WANT YOU TO LOVE ME." If we examine the sentence I WANT YOU TO LOVE ME in greater detail, it becomes evident that the subject *I* and object *You* contain multiple realities. Consider the *I* who is the patient. The *I* who wants me to love her may refer to the patient in actuality, that is, as she is today; let us call this *I Ms. X*. The *I* may, in addition, refer to another level of reality—not the Ms. X as she is in ordinary life but the Ms. X who is my patient; that is, Ms. X within the frame of the psychoanalytic setting. In this case we will refer to her as analysand X. Or the *I* may be a reference to the little girl in Ms. X, perhaps both the preadolescent who felt loved by her father and the adolescent who was rejected by him. At this level of reality let us say that this *I* = *daughter*.

Now let us consider the object of her love, the *You* in this sentence. This *You* could refer to me as an ordinary man, as someone perceived outside of my professional imago or role. Let us leave aside for the moment the fact that, like Calvino's author, I may be choosing to present only certain facets of myself. The *You* in the sentence may also refer to another level of reality: that of the analyst functioning within the frame. There is yet a third level of reality, that of the iconic/projective transference. At this "iconic" level of reality, *You* = *father*. There is a further question: am I her early loving father, her later rejecting father, or the father that is about to be lost?

In the sentence I WANT YOU TO LOVE ME, we must now consider the *Me*. Who is the *Me* demanding to be loved? Is it the young married woman who is seeking love? Is it the analysand who is seeking to be loved? Or is it the daughter who is seeking the love that she had lost? This *Me* can also represent at least three different levels of reality: Ms. X in ordinary life; Ms. X as a patient; Ms. X as a daughter.

This can be represented schematically as follows:

	WANT	TO LOVE		
I	YOU	ME	LEVEL OF REALITY
Ms. X	A.H.M.	Ms. X	Ordinary life
Analysand X	Dr. A.H.M.	Analysand X	Dependent/Containing
Daughter	Father	Daughter	Iconic/Projective transference

Given the existence of multiple aspects of the self and object combined with the multiple levels of reality present within the consulting room, it is understandable that the transference creates insoluble dilemmas and paradoxes. In this illustration the patient's dilemmas are manifold: her love is impossible to gratify since the object of her love exists in different levels of reality. Gratification at any one level of reality leads to paradoxical frustration at another. If she did experience love from me as a "real" object, this would disrupt the frame of the analysis; she would in effect lose the analysis. If I interpreted her wish to be loved by me as *only* a displacement of her wish to be loved by her father, she might feel that such an observation was demeaning and rejecting, as if I were saying that this is *only* a transference reaction. If she experienced love from me as a father, she would then be confronted with an acute sense of loss because she would have to acknowledge that her relation with her father was irretrievably gone, and thus the experience of transference love would evoke mourning.

Despite the complexities of the illustration just presented, it is possible to discern distinct, separate levels of reality as in Calvino's example of *A Midsummer Night's Dream*. In this illustration, at least three levels of reality are present in the consulting room: (1) that of ordinary life; (2) the level of reality contained within the frame; (3) that of the "father," iconic transference. With regard to level (1), I am reminded of Anna Freud's statement: "I feel still that we should leave room somewhere for the realization that analyst and patient are also two real people, of equal adult status, in a real personal relationship to each other" (cited in Greenson and Wexler 1969, p. 27). The third level of reality is the recreation within the transference of specific elements in the patient's relationship with her father, who had been loving in early childhood, then withdrawn and depressed in her adolescence, and who had died before anything could be resolved. These levels of reality are separate, as are the sense of self and object.

The Transference Neurosis: An Obsolete Concept

There is great confusion surrounding the term *transference neurosis* (see Panel 1987; Reed 1987; Cooper 1987; London 1987). It has been used in two contexts: in the first, the term is a marker in a nosological sense to separate the "classical" neuroses from the so-called narcissistic disorders. But inasmuch as the centrality of the Oedipus complex already defines the classical case, such a definition is redundant if not tautological. A second context is Freud's reference to the transference neurosis as an artificial illness in which the analysand's "infantile" neurosis is recreated as a fresh illness in relation to the analyst. This definition has since been eroded by many factors: some patients have never experienced a symptomatic "infantile" neurosis (A. Freud 1971). Further, Glover (1955, p. 123) notes that the transference neurosis may be in the category of a pseudo-scientific slogan: "The term *transference neurosis* with all its theoretical and practical implications has fallen into relative desuetude." Glover goes on to say that the transference neurosis is not infrequently absent, and in the average opening phase signs of transference are unobtrusive and fleeting. Finally, it should be noted that the entire issue of the transference neurosis has become politicized. Some analysts believe that the transference neurosis is absent in other forms of psychotherapy, so that its presence is taken to be the hallmark of psychoanalysis (Blum 1971). Reed (1987) observes that there is, for this reason, a political stake in finding the transference neurosis, and thus its observation in a psychoanalytic case does not rule out the influence of the analyst's suggestion. After a thoughtful review of the current and past literature concerning the transference neurosis, Cooper (1987) concludes: "Our search seems to lead to the painful conclusion that the concept of the transference neurosis has lost its specificity and efforts to clarify it no longer expand our vision. The concept should be abandoned." I share in his opinion.

Because the essential paradox of transference was not identified by Freud, it was possible for two such distinguished analysts as Anna

Freud and Hans Loewald, who both believed themselves to be extending Freud's view of transference, to hold opposite opinions. Loewald (1980) believed that the term *transference neurosis* should be restricted to the *new* creation that arises out of the analytic work and should not refer to the automatic repetition of the old illness. Anna Freud, in her most significant work, *The Ego and the Mechanisms of Defense,* defined transference in a precisely opposite fashion (1936, p. 18): "By transference we mean all those impulses experienced by the patient in his relation with the analyst *which are not newly created* by the objective analytic situation but have their source in early—indeed, the very earliest—object relations and are now merely revived under the influence of the repetition compulsion" (my emphasis).

The following passage suggests that Freud may have sensed the paradox of the many levels of reality represented by transference without making it explicit (Freud 1914, p. 154):[4]

> The main instrument, however, for curbing the patient's compulsion to repeat and for turning it into a motive for remembering lies in the handling of the transference. We render the compulsion harmless, and indeed useful, by giving it the right to assert itself in a definite field. *We admit it into the transference as a playground in which it is allowed to expand in almost complete freedom . . .* we regularly succeed in giving all the symptoms of the illness a new transference meaning and in replacing his ordinary neurosis by a "transference neurosis" of which he can be cured by the therapeutic work. *The transference thus creates an intermediate region between illness and real life through which the transition from the one to the other is made* [my emphasis].

Freud's reference to a playground, to an intermediate region between illness and real life, is suggestive of a description of another level of reality. But this is only an intimation that he never developed further. Despite the importance of the subject, Freud added hardly anything more to his discussion of transference after his early papers on technique.

Confusion of Levels of Reality: Projective Identification

A young single woman who was withdrawn and depressed complained that I was not helping her in her treatment because I was not making useful comments and interpretations. I, in turn, was feeling frustrated because I felt that in her withdrawn, mostly silent, unengaged state, it was not possible to say anything that was meaningful. In response to her complaint, I did say that she wanted me to produce something "out of the blue." I do not know why I chose that particular expression, but, much to my surprise, it evoked an intense reaction of rage. My experience was one of being attacked for making an "innocent" remark; her attack on me felt "out of the blue." The meaning of this particular interaction became clearer sometime later. The patient had a dream about "booby traps," which we could trace to her experience with her father. The metaphor of the booby trap was particularly apt, since a booby trap can be an innocuous object which, if touched, could set off an unexpected and disastrous explosion. Her father was in this sense "booby-trapped" in that the patient had had the experience of making what appeared to be an innocuous remark which would set off an inexplicable rage. I cannot say whether my choice of the expression "out of the blue" was chance or whether it was unconsciously determined, for I did have a sense from prior experience that our relationship might be "booby-trapped." But her reaction is undoubtedly testimony to the evocative power of language.

This small slice of transference interaction contrasts with the description of the transference in the previous illustration in that here levels of reality are not separated, but the affective memories that comprise inner reality have been displaced into the analyst. I experienced quite directly what the patient had felt in her interaction with her father. This could be described as a *projective identification*. By means of empathy, we ordinarily enter into another's psychic reality. But empathy is a voluntary act, whereas projective identification is involuntary for both the recipient of the projections and the person from whom these projections originate. Moreover, in this process there is not simply a reversal of roles, for the patient also felt attacked by me, so that we *both* were attacker and attacked. In this confusion there was not a loss of identity: I experienced what the patient had experienced as a child, but there was no sense of merging identities; we both retained a sense of ourselves. What was projected was an encapsulated, specific affective experience—a sector or slice of the analysand's inner or psychic reality.

In this transference interaction, although the patient was intensely angry, she was also aware of a wish to be held and loved by me. Thus another sector of reality was also present, recreating a very different relationship with her father. At this other level of reality the experience was that of reaching out in love only to be rebuffed and rejected. This sector was also projected into me in that I had the repeated experience of reaching out to be helpful only to find my positive efforts somehow turned into the opposite.[5] For example, the patient asked during a session in which she was very withdrawn and silent whether I was feeling bored. Previously I had sidestepped such questions, but I now felt that our relationship was sufficiently secure that I could respond to her question in a more direct fashion. I also hoped that a more direct acknowledgment of her need to withdraw might help her to have more control over this distressing symptom. I accordingly said that, yes, I was bored, but that my boredom was not a rejection of her but a response to her withdrawal. I said further that I knew this to be something that she needed to do; I wished to convey to her that I was not being critical of the fact that she was withdrawn but was trying to understand why she needed to do so at this particular time. It should also be noted that I knew this patient had read some of my publications on the subject of the use of boredom as a countertransference response. Thus there was also something collegial in my response, which proved to be a misjudgment, in that I mistakenly judged the patient to be in a more mature position than she actually was. This error in clinical judgment no doubt represented a wish: my collegial response was experienced as a rejection of her dependency. The patient reacted angrily: she did experience my comment that I was bored as a rejection of her; she felt that I did not understand her, that I was out of synchrony with her, and so forth. I, in turn, felt that I had responded to her in a caring fashion, and that by admitting my boredom I was acknowledging the healthier, more "mature" side of her personality. In this she was correct in judging that I was out of synchrony with her. My reaction to her anger recreated in me precisely what she had repeatedly feared and anticipated with her father: that attempting to draw closer to another person evokes an unexpected, angry rejection—in short, that one's love is dangerous.

The experiencing of a projective identification can be said to rupture the frame of the analytic setting; it can also be viewed as a confusion of the multiple levels of reality present in the therapeutic process. It would be inaccurate to describe this process as a loss of the boundaries of personal identity; this simply did not occur in the illustration I just gave. What was confusing was not the loss of identity but the experiencing of someone else's psychic reality. This results in a temporary rupture of the frame, with a consequent loss of this level of reality, the reality of the therapeutic setting—a reality separate from that of ordinary life.

Projective identification is a form of defense, in which painful, unwanted portions of the self are projected into the object. It is also a form of communication. I believe it to be a widespread phenomenon and not something that is present only in severe psychopathology. The process of entering into the psychic reality of another person is portrayed in literature and myth, especially in Eastern cultures. For example, entering into someone else's reality or sharing a common psychic reality is a recurrent theme in Indian mythology (O'Flaherty 1984), as in stories in which lovers, unknown to each other, dream the same dream and subsequently find each other in waking life. Another variant of the shared reality is the Indian myth that the narrative of our lives is nothing more than the dreams of a God. Melanie Klein (1963), who was the first to observe projective identification, illustrated the phenomenon by referring to the novel *If I Were You* by the French novelist Julian Green. Fabian, the hero of the novel, makes a pact with the devil that enables him to change himself into other people. The Devil teaches Fabian a magic formula which includes his own name, for it is of the utmost importance that he not forget his own name. In this way Fabian enters into the reality of another but preserves his own identity.

Woody Allen, who is no stranger to psychoanalysis, used this same theme of entering into other realities in the movie *The Purple Rose of Cairo*, in which the hero of the film leaves the screen and enters into the life of a woman in the audience. Woody Allen is also associated with the following joke that illustrates the entry into someone else's reality: First man: "I need to take my brother to a psychiatrist because he thinks that he is a chicken." Second man: "Why don't you take him to a psychiatrist?" First man: "I can't because we need the eggs."

When the analysand projects his inner life into the analyst, it is as if the analyst is an actor who receives stage directions from the patient, but the entire process remains outside the consciousness of both participants. For some patients it seems that their affective experiences need to be placed within the other because language itself is inadequate, and some other means must be found to communicate.

The following is an example of projective identification observed in the supervision of a female analyst. A male analysand who experienced his mother as manipulative, sexually overstimulating, and demeaning placed this experience within his analyst in the following fashion: on one occasion when he followed behind her into the consulting room, he told her that he wished to rape her. The intensity and immediacy of this statement were such that the analyst found it to be quite unnerving. In this fashion the analyst was forced to enter into the patient's psychic reality as she experienced a sexual stimulation that was frightening, inappropriate, and demeaning. The analyst was made to feel precisely what the patient had experienced with his mother.

As Calvino observed with regard to literature, levels of reality may be kept separate, as in *A Midsummer Night's Dream,* or may melt and mingle together, as in *Hamlet.* Projective identification illustrates the latter condition. The problem is further complicated by the fact that the term *reality* refers both to *levels* of reality and to the *construction* of reality. I have been using the term *levels of reality* to refer to the distinction between ordinary life, the frame of the analysis, and the iconic transformations. But in addition to these different levels of reality, the phenomenon of projective identification includes a confusion of the constructed realities of subject and object. This quickly leads to the question: whose (internal) reality is it? In projective identification the internal reality of the subject is projected into the object, resulting in a confused mingling and involuntary sharing of these two different levels of reality. This naturally leads to a disruption of the frame since the analyst can no longer be perceived as within the frame by the analysand, and the analyst also for a period of time may not function as an analyst.

Melanie Klein viewed the concept of projective identification primarily as a defense in association with her theory of the paranoid position, where, under pressure from the death instinct, the infant projects part of the self sadistically into the interior of the mother's body in order to control the mother from within (Segal 1981). From the standpoint of an outside observer, this process could be described as the child's fantasy. But I wonder whether it is true that the experience of projective identification is articulated as a fantasy. My observations of adult patients who are experiencing a projective identification do not provide any indication that they are having a fantasy of entering into the body or the psychic space of the analyst. To describe projective identification as a fantasy is a post hoc reconstruction from the standpoint of a detached observer, an attempt to view a some-what mysterious and inexplicable process as if it were a narrative. The fact that projective identification has mistakenly been classified under the heading of a fantasy has resulted in the valid criticism that the concept confuses fantasy and process.[6] Since this term was introduced by Melanie Klein, the concept of projective identification has undergone a continuous process of evolution (see Sandler 1987 for a succinct presentation of this process). The fact that projective identification takes place involuntarily on the part of the analysand is consistent with its defensive nature; it is an automatic involuntary action analogous to the automatic physiological defenses of the body.

In Bion's hands (1962), the term *projective identification* underwent a change of meaning, with the defensive, intrapsychic (one-person psychology) aspect de-emphasized. The concept was placed firmly within the context of a two-person psychology in that projective identification was now understood to be an early or primitive form of the child's communicating anxiety to the mother in order for the anxiety to be contained or predigested and then returned. The mother, if she is functioning well enough, reflects the noxious affects back into the child in a detoxified form. The communication of affects is a form of action involving both mother and child, with the mother acting as a container for what needs to be contained. Couched in the language of that period of development, Bion's description of this process (1962, p. 7) refers to an "evacuation" of psychic pain that is then "digested" by the mother. Shifting from an alimentary to an anal metaphor, Meltzer (1967) extended Bion's ideas to describe the mother as a "toilet-breast."

When projective identification is observed in the psychoanalysis of adult patients, it is not only the "noxious" affects that need to be contained; what is projected into the analyst may present an entire interactive scenario. A sector of an internalized drama centered upon a core of affects (in the next chapter I will describe this as an *affect category*) is projected into the analyst. Frequently, but not invariably, there is a reversal of roles: the victimized patient becomes the aggressor and the analyst becomes the victim.[7] This record of traumatic interactions with parental caretakers may or may not be veridical, but it does correspond to a level of psychic reality. When the patient's psychic reality enters into the experience of the analyst, there is, as I have mentioned, a loss on the patient's part, and perhaps on the analyst's as well, of the apperception of the multiple *separate* levels of reality present in the therapeutic setup. This form of transference, therefore, is one in which the separateness of levels of reality is not preserved; this is another way of describing the absence of a therapeutic alliance. (This subject will be discussed further in Chapter 8.)

Interpretation, if successful, restores the frame of the therapeutic or psychoanalytic setting. Interpretation can only occur, however, after the analyst has restored the separateness of his or her inner reality and is able to use the projective identification as the patient's communication. This constructive use of the countertransference is due in no small measure to the pioneering contributions of Heimann (1950) and Racker (1968). We also know, however, that projective identifications can become a persistent and chronic form of communication between analyst and analysand, especially if the analyst has not been able to separate her own psychic reality from that of the analysand. Baranger and colleagues (1983) have referred to the stalemating of the transference/countertransference as a "bastion."

Although projective identification may be regarded as a primitive form of communication, it is present in transference/countertransference interactions to a greater degree than has been recognized. Experiencing multiple levels of current and archaic realities is both a repetition of the past and a recontextualization of that experience in current time. The problem of transference repetition and the experience of time will be considered in the following two chapters.

4

Repetition and Retranscription

Freud's theory of the repetition compulsion required the postulation of a natural force that transcended the evident desire of all sentient beings to seek pleasure and to avoid pain. Freud believed that the death instinct was such a force. But contemporary biology offers no evidence that would support Freud's theorizing. Freud was not incorrect, however, in judging repetition to be a fundamental biological phenomenon. Although his psychobiology is no longer credible, it is not dissimilar to other sweeping scientific theories that characterized the late nineteenth century.

An alternative psychobiological explanation of the repetition compulsion has recently been proposed by Gerald Edelman (1987). As noted earlier, in his book *Neural Darwinism* he revolutionizes the theory of memory by proposing that memory does not consist of a permanent record in the brain that is isomorphic with past experience, but rather that memory is a dynamic reconstruction that is context-bound and established by means of categories. This description of memory is fully consistent with and provides a neurobiological backing for Freud's concept of *Nachträglichkeit*. Edelman's new theory of memory, perception, and cognition offers an alternative explanation for the repetition of that which is painful inasmuch as the refinding of perceptual categories transcends the seeking of pleasure. In this theory the motoric system plays a vital part in perception, from which it can be inferred that the repetitive affects of transference function similarly to categorical memories. Transference affects are motoric in that they actively scan the human environment in order to refind an affective category. This scanning, as we know, not only may be a refinding but also may lead to a self-fulfilling prophecy to the extent that transference affects induce a complementary counter-transference response. *Thus, the repetition of painful affect categories is an essential mode of cognition. In this process the patient's motor apparatus (affects) evokes the therapist's affective responses to find a perceptual "fit," to establish an affect category.*

The evocation of countertransference affects can also be viewed as a form of affect training in that the affective responses of the therapist are enlisted both to confirm and to disconfirm affect categories. The patient's use of the analyst's affective responses may also be placed in the service of repairing developmental deficits in that the analyst's affective responses may lead to a *replacement* for that which was missing.

Neurobiology and the Repetition Compulsion

Transference repetition appears at first as evidence of yet another transference paradox, for endless repetition of behavior can lead to a cul-de-sac; yet transference repetition is the means, and perhaps the only means, of effecting therapeutic change. Transference repetition has long been understood to be both a resistance to change and the motor that drives therapeutic change. The compulsion to repeat can be seen as something that can only be passively endured, as one's fate is passively endured, or it can be viewed as an attempt to achieve *active mastery.*

The repetitive actions expressed in the transference were seen by Freud as an alternative to remembering, that is, an "inferior" form of remembering indicating the strength of the resistance: "The greater the resistance, the more extensively will acting out (repetition) replace remembering" (1914, p. 151). In judging repetitive actions to be an inferior form of remembering as compared to verbalization, Freud was probably thinking of hypnosis, in which remembering the content held under repression removed the symptom. Yet Freud recognized that it was only by means of transference repetition, a form of action, that the curative process took place. The patient's illness must be recreated "not as an event in the past but as a present-day force" (p. 151), and "when all is said and done, it is impossible to destroy anyone *in absentia or in effigy*" (1912, p. 108).

Almost all considerations of the subject of repetition and the repetition compulsion recognize this paradoxical aspect of transference—

that the transference transposes categories from the past into the present, yet the relation to the analyst is a new object relationship. Loewald stated (1980, p. 89) that "repetition means possible novel configurations and novel resolutions of the conflict."

Freud believed that repetition within the transference was one of the few direct expressions of an otherwise silent death instinct. For Freud, the death instinct moved mutely as a fundamental inertia in living systems, an urge inherent in organic life to return to an earlier state of things, displaying a demonic quality in its disregard of plea- sure. How then can this blind, destructive compulsion to repeat also be the means through which new learning is acquired? Blind repetition does not allow for learning, as it does not allow for novelty or for the unexpected. Freud's preoccupation with his speculative psychobiology during this particular stage in his life led to a certain disparity between his clinically accurate description of repetitive phe- nomena and his broad, if not wild, speculations concerning the death instinct. Accordingly, the essay "Beyond the Pleasure Principle" (Freud 1920a) is divided into two portions: a clincial introduction that includes the description of the repetitive action of a child's game, and a very abstract discussion influenced by late nineteenth-century psychophysics. Freud describes a child who, by means of a mimetic act, masters the pain of his mother's departure by throwing and retrieving a spool over the side of his cot. This child's game illustrates the view that the repetition compulsion is not a passively endured death instinct but represents a form of symbolic *action*. The child succeeds in mastering the trauma of his mother's departure by a symbolic repetition, a game that creates the illusion of a separate reality in which the trauma of the "real" or ordinary world is re- moved into the internal world. Winnicott would later describe this as "bringing trauma within the orbit of personal omnipotence."

In this focus on the inevitability of repetition in linear time, Freud apparently forgot or put aside his earlier ideas concerning *Nachträg- lichkeit*. Laplanche and Pontalis (1973) observe that Freud never clearly defined this term, although it was indisputably part of his intellectual equipment. *Nachträglichkeit* refers to traumatic or unas- similated memories that are later revised—a view that is fully consis- tent with the "working through" in the transference of the memory of an experience that had been traumatic, incomplete, or unassimilated. However, Edelman's theory suggests that *Nachträglichkeit*, as evidenced in human psychology, is a special or restricted illustration of a universal characteristic of the nervous system to establish perceptual identities of categorical memories.

The hedonic or pleasure principle, that an organism seeks pleasure and avoids pain, appears to be self-evident and commonsensical. If one reasons teleologically, this pleasure principle must be based upon a fundamental property of animal life. If an organism is motivated by something that supersedes, takes precedence over, and goes beyond pleasure, Freud rightly assumed that another equally powerful biological force must exist to counterbalance the pleasure motive. It was necessary for Freud, then, to view the death instinct as equally powerful and equally ubiquitous, as something that represented a fundamental biological principle.

According to Edelman's theory propounded in *Neural Darwinism*, cognitive repetition through the recreation of categorical memory is also a fundamental biological principle. His theory is also a theory of repetition that supersedes the pleasure principle, but unlike Freud's biological speculations, it is the product of the current revolution in the neurosciences. He approaches the problem from a very different direction, from that of a theory of cognition. The commonsensical and traditional view that the motor systems and the sensory and perceptual systems operate sequentially is incorrect and misleading. In the traditional view, perception activates a motoric response. A more accurate view is that motoric activity is essential for perception and learning; the motoric response is an integral part of perception. The motor end of the central nervous system provides a continual testing of new environments that is essential for the perception of categories. A central tenet of Edelman's theory is that perception is a rediscovery, a refinding of categories held in memory. Freud also suggested in his paper "Negation" (1925) that the aim of reality testing is not to find an object in real perception that corresponds to the one presented, but *to refind such an object*. Freud also viewed perception as an active process (1925, p. 238): "For, in our hypothesis, perception is not a purely passive process. The ego periodically sends out small amounts of cathexis into the perceptual system, by means of which it samples the external stimuli, and then after every such tentative advance it draws back again."

The compulsion to repeat represents a compulsion to seek a perceptual identity between present and past objects. The refinding of categories stored in memory at first appears to be a high-level mental function associated with language, but Edelman assembled evidence suggesting that categorical memory exists in lower animals, such as pigeons, who do not possess language but demonstrate startling capacities for perceptual generalizations. Thus he proposes that the refinding of categories represents a transcendent property of the central nervous system. Edelman's theory not only provides a more plausible alternative to the death instinct but also resolves the apparent paradox of how repetition can result in new experiences and learning.

To summarize the relevant elements of Edelman's theory: motoric action is essential for perception; perception consists of the refinding of categories held in memory; this refinding requires repetitive action during which the environment, as Freud also observed, is periodically sampled and tested so that when novelty is encountered there is a *retranscription* of memory in a new context. Edelman's theory is a revolutionary view of memory in that memory is no longer seen as a passive registration of experience in which there is an isomorphic correspondence between the event and the memory trace. What is stored in memory is not a replica of the event, but rather the *potential* to generalize or refind the category or class of which the event is a member. "Recategorical memory is dynamic, transformational, associative, and distributed—its procedures are *representative* of categorizations, but are not necessarily representations" (Edelman 1987, p. 270). If categories are seen as the basic element of thought, this is consistent with the observation that thinking in metaphor, a categorical form of thinking, is the currency of the mind.

As noted earlier, Edelman's theory of memory as the retranscription of categories was intuitively anticipated by Freud in his concept of *Nachträglichkeit*. There are, however, significant differences between Freud and Edelman in that Freud did not recognize that memory consisted of the refinding of categories, and he believed in the existence of permanent memory traces. But a belief in permanent memory, which is stored by means of some form of neuronal or synaptic alteration that is isomorphic with experience, was a widely held assumption until Edelman's recent and still controversial challenge.[1]

Affect Categories in the Transference and Countertransference

Transference repetition can now be viewed as a special class of perceptual retranscriptions. Transference is a mode of perception in which an old category is imposed on a current or new object, creating the compulsion to seek a perceptual identity between the past and the present. For this reason, transference has always been recognized as something that is not limited to the treatment situation. It is a refinding in the present of a category from the past which may or may not prove to be a categorical fit; it is the imposition of an internal template upon what is presented from without. Transference repetition, unlike learning in general, is a response to the pressure of unassimilated experience. Experiences may be unassimilated because of trauma or because of the absence of something from the environment that was needed at a nodal point in development. The difference between transference phenomena within the treatment situation and transference as it occurs in life itself is that *the treatment setup is designed to accentuate multiple levels of reality, which in turn enlarges the potential for both old perceptions and retranscriptions of new perceptions.* In Edelman's theory of memory, action is essential for perception. Affective expression is the motoric action of transference; affects are the action element in transference that bring the memory of past experiences into the present. Freud's distinction between the fate of affects and the verbal presentations of the preconscious system[2] may have obscured the fact that affects are never content-free.[3]

The concept of *affect categories* approaches familiar observations from a somewhat different perspective. Edelman's theory provides a biological backing for the old term *complex,* which can now be reexamined in terms of affect categories. The assumption is that affective experience and affectively charged fantasies are stored in a manner that is analogous to categorical memory. Such affect categories exist as a *potential* awaiting activation in current experience. To the extent that a given affect category represents unassimilated trauma, or a central pathogenic fantasy, there will be a pressure to evoke a corresponding countertransference affective response in the other person that will be self-confirming. One may think of the environmental stimulus that releases such affective categories as similar to Proust's tasting a crumb of madeleine, which released the recollection of his childhood. Certain intense affect states create their own releasing stimuli by means of the communicative function of affects that creates a corresponding affect state in the object. Where intense countertransference affects are evoked, as in projective identification, a perceptual identity between past and present is created by the patient. It is in this way that repetition of affects is a self-fulfilling prophecy.

The Oedipus complex, from this point of view, has the potential to evoke a multitude of incongruous and conflicting affect categories. If we think of the specific affect categories evoked by the positive and the negative Oedipus complex, which consist of a congeries of both experiences and fantasies,[4] we have a picture of the complexity of the affect categories that can be recreated in a thorough psychoanalysis with respect to a particular phase of development. To this we must add the re-evocation of earlier unassimilated experience, which also includes former loving relationships that were superseded by a later negative development.

Affect categories reflect the memory of a unique constellation of experience (whether veridical or not); they can be thought of as units of experience of the past brought into present time. Affect categories may or may not contribute to ego structures. Fairbairn (1952) introduced the idea that unassimilated interactive experiences between the child and his caretakers were internalized as ego structures (internalized objects). In this sense Fairbairn's theory of internal objects bears some relation to the concept of affect categories, but not all affect categories result in a deformation of the ego, as my clinical vignettes will illustrate.

The memories of affective experiences are organized into categories as an attempt to find a perceptual unity between past and present. Affect categories concerning the self, or the self in relation to objects, can be observed most clearly in the process of projective identification. There, as illustrated in the previous chapter, specific and multiple affect categories from the patient's past are "placed" into the therapist.

The refinding of archaic affect categories in present time is, then, a basis mode of cognition. When the archaic affect category predominates over current perceptions, it may contribute to the psychopathology of everyday life. For example, a patient reported the following incident: because his airline went on strike, my patient was stranded in a distant city and unable to return home. He did everything possible to obtain passage on another airline: he cajoled and pleaded with the functionaries of other airlines, all to no avail. Although my patient was usually not unduly anxious and was in fact a highly experienced traveler, who in the past had remained calm under circumstances that would frighten many people, in this particular situation he experienced an overwhelming and generalized panic. He felt as if the unyielding airline representatives were like Nazis, and the underground passages of the airline terminal resembled a concentration camp. The helplessness of not being able to return home, combined with the institutional intransigence of the authorities, evoked the following affect category. When this man was three years old, he and his parents, Jewish residents of a central European country, were desperately attempting to escape from the Nazis. They did in fact manage to obtain an airline passage to freedom, but until that point the outcome was very much in doubt. Although my patient did not recall his affective state at that time, his parents reported that he had seemed cheerful and unaffected by their great anxiety. In this example, his helpless inability to leave a foreign city together with the intransigence of the authorities evoked a specific affect category that remained as a potential memory of an unassimilated past experience.

Another patient reacted with anxiety and rage when he discovered that the woman whom he loved and with whom he was living was on one occasion drunk. The affective category evoked was that of emotional absence, since his mother had not been "there" for him as a child. But the affective reaction, although derived from his relation to his mother, took on, as it were, a life of its own; it was perceived as an entity, as a category of experience—a reaction of anger and anxiety when the other person is not "there." Similarly, another man whose mother had been psychotic during his childhood reacted with anxiety to minimal signs of unreliability in his wife: unreliability evoked the category of his sterotypic response to his psychotic mother.

Affect categories are also derived from the self, taken as an object. Induction of negative countertransference affects may represent the activation of a specific category of self-hatred. Through the process of projective identification, the therapist may be induced to feel precisely that same complex of feelings that the patient experienced toward herself.[5] For example, the patient may successfully induce an attitude in the therapist that replicates her worst fears. It is as if the patient's "badness" has been exteriorized through the communication of a specific affect category. In this fashion I have experienced analysands as "destructive," "borderline," "empty," "superficial," "incapable of loving," and so forth. In such cases it seems that the patient needs to enlist the analyst's affective response to find a perceptual identity, to confirm a category of self-perception. Behind the compulsion to repeat, there is also a wish by the patient to have her perception disconfirmed. When the analyst succeeds in recognizing this process as a projective identification, interpretation may result in a disconfirmation of a particular affect category. It is in this sense that affects, part of the motor apparatus, are used for cognition. The process of *disconfirmation* is essentially a process of *retranscription*.

Freud was not mistaken in viewing affects as part of the motor apparatus, but he could not know that motoric action was essential for perception. He chose to illustrate affect "discharge" by referring to dreams in which affects are "discharged" into the interior of the mental apparatus (Freud 1915). But the state of dreaming is a special instance in which the individual is cut off from the external world. If Freud had realized that motoric action of affects is one of the means through which the ego actively tests the human environment, he could not have continued to subscribe to a "discharge" theory of affects. In waking life, affects are communicative and contagious, so that the other person is involved in the affective repetition and will collude, either consciously or unconsciously, in confirming or disconfirming the subject's category of perception.

Affective categories may be thought of as units of perception within each individual's private world, so that with the evocation of the *other's* response, there is the possibility of a novel perception and hence of learning from experience. The patient's rejection of the analyst's novel affective response, or failure to perceive that response, comes under the heading of resistance, which will be considered in Chapter 7.

Russell (1985) introduced the very useful idea of *affective competence*—that affect repetitions can be thought of as analogous to the development of a motor skill. For example, a male analysand during the first several years of his analysis disagreed with nearly everything that I said. Moreover, he never failed to seize upon anything for which I could be justifiably criticized. His affective position and the counter-response aroused in me could be described as combative. This affective repetition could be understood, in one sense, as a "training for masculinity"; his combativeness was a test of masculine courage. To beard the lion in his den is to act like a man, to act like the patient's father, who was in fact particularly courageous during World War II. It will come as no surprise that this combative masculinity was a defense against an opposite trait: in another sector of his personality this patient identified himself as a submissive, passive woman whose autonomy would be not respected. I was enlisted as his sparring partner in this lesson in affect training. The fact that the analysis proceeded in spite of the combat and that we both survived was enormously reassuring to the patient. This may illustrate the therapeutic value of reaching what Winnicott (1971) called the point of maximum destructiveness, which he believed to be, at a deeper level, an affirmation of externality and separateness.

It is evident that the therapist is enlisted as a necessary collaborator in the process of affect training, or to put it more accurately, affect retraining. The content of the affect categories that are recreated in this collaborative exchange between patient and therapist is naturally quite variegated, but nevertheless we can discuss two broad classes: one is a repetition of what has been experienced in the past, and the other is a search for what should have occurred but did not occur— an attempt to redress an absence or a deficit. It is probable that there is also a potential to repeat what did *not happen*. We may think of this as a negative affect category, which also may prove to be self-confirming in the induction of a complementary absence in the analyst.

These affect categories include not only stereotypical reactions to objects but also, as noted, the recreation of archaic feelings of love and hatred regarding the self taken as an object. I have described the projection of self-hatred resulting in a corresponding negative countertransference. Kohut (1977), on the other hand, has emphasized the projection of what might be described as the beloved or idealized self.[6] Affects associated with an idealized or grandiose self may be "placed" in the therapist to form what has been called the idealizing transference. Thus, affect categories in relation to the self are treated no differently from those in relation to other persons: in both instances there is a compulsion to repeat and to reaffirm a perceptual identity and to enlist the other person in testing those perceptions. The hated aspect of the self may be a shell that protects a hidden, beloved sense of self, as in Winnicott's distinction between the true and the false self. Patients will then use the therapist's affective responses as a means of defensively re-establishing the false self, with the unexpressed hope that the therapist in her affective responses will interrupt this repetitive confirmation of archaic affect categories.

A female analyst observed that her patient, a young woman, had developed a persistent and obnoxious body odor. When the analyst finally felt able to introduce this delicate matter into the analysis, it was subsequently learned that not only did the patient consider herself to be disgusting and dirty but she believed that her mother also considered her to be disgusting and dirty, since when the patient was being toilet-trained her mother was repulsed by her "messes." This entire complex of affective responses was revived in the transference/ countertransference for the simple reason that the patient had, without thinking about it, stopped washing during this phase of her analysis. As the analyst was able to analyze her own countertransference she was able to interpret to the patient the meaning behind her compulsion to present herself as a repulsive person. The patient initially enlisted the analyst in a collusive reaffirmation of archaic affect categories. The analyst's affective responses at first repeated the mother's response, reaffirming that particular archaic affect category. But as the analyst was able to analyze her own affective responses, she could then interrupt and disconfirm the repetition by means of an interpretation.

The Analyst's Response to the Patient's Affect Deficits

Individual differences regarding the capacity to tolerate affects have long been recognized as an attribute of temperament. The extent to which temperament itself is a fixed genetic trait and the extent to which it can be modified by experience remains an open question. Greenacre (1953) believed that an individual's predisposition to anxiety may have originated as a result of trauma in the earliest developmental period, including the experience of birth. Zetzel (1949) recognized that being able to tolerate depression is a prognostic indicator of the suitability for psychoanalysis. The capacity to tolerate affects such as depression and anxiety was seen by Zetzel as necessary for normal maturation; as a corollary, affect intolerance is a contributing factor in states of ego defect or deficit. It is reasonable to suppose that such a trait or predisposition can be modified by the affective responses of the child's caretakers, by the ability of the caretaker to contain the child's affects; an anxious child raised by an anxious mother will certainly be different from an anxious child raised by a calm mother. I return here to Bion's theory of the container and the contained.

Low affect tolerance may lead to projective identification, which, in addition to its defensive and communicative functions, can also be used as a means of affect retraining. There is an evident advantage if a patient can project affects outside of the self so that they can be treated as something external; without this projection, the patient is helpless and cannot escape from what he is feeling. If affects can be displaced or externalized into someone else, they can then be treated as an object in the environment.

In the repetition or refinding of affect categories there may be no fundamental distinction between the refinding of a memory, whether veridical or not, and the search for an experience that never happened. In the latter case the patient does not project a specific schema upon the analyst but rather enlists the analyst to collude in a repetition of what was missing. Such experiences have a more diffuse character, a nonspecificity that is consistent with the recreation of a developmental absence.

The repetitive search for an experience that never happened, the search for what was absent, also evokes the analyst's affective responses. Here the analyst's affective response is not as immediate and intense as is the countertransference reponse to a projective identification. In Chapter 2 I described how the analyst's metacommunications, which include the communication of affects, are utilized symbolically to actualize developmental conflicts. There I focused particularly on conflicts concerning autonomy and separateness; I also described how the analyst's actions, as an analyst, are transformed into a dependent/containing transference. The inclusion of the term *containing* emphasizes the significance of the analyst's capacity to contain the analysand's affects, a view that is consistent with Bion's theory of the container and the contained. In this section I plan to describe in further detail how the patient may use the analyst's or therapist's affective responses to alleviate deficiencies.

Not only does the mother contain the child's affects, but she also, in her mirror response, identifies the child's affects. Daniel Stern (1985) introduced the term *affect attunement,* which appears to be synonymous with the mirror response. Stern observed from the direct observation of mothers and their infants that mothers match the infant's state of feeling not necessarily by imitating the infant but by conveying, often symbolically, that there has been a recognition of the infant's affect state. For example, Stern describes the following interaction (1985, p. 140): "A nine-month-old girl becomes very excited about a toy and reaches for it. As she grabs it, she lets out an exuberant 'aaaah!' and looks at her mother. Her mother looks back, scrunches up her shoulders, and performs a terrific shimmy with the upper body, like a go-go dancer. The shimmy lasts only about as long

as her daughter's 'aaaah!' but is equally excited, joyful, and intense."
Stern notes that the important thing about the mother's affective
response is that it is spontaneous and automatic, and occurs largely
outside of her awareness. I would add that the mother's normative
reaction reinforces and confirms the *perceptual* validity of the child's
affective response.

It is reasonable to believe that mothers who are unable to respond
in this way to their child's affective states, as Stern has so well described, will contribute to a deficiency in the child's capacity to identify, accept, and contain her own affects. This maternal inability, often
described as lack of *empathy,* will contribute to this specific developmental deficiency. I shall further assume that such a child will, during
later life, continue to have difficulty in identifying and accepting her
own affective experiences. In the therapeutic setting, such individuals
will enlist the therapist in the process of identifying their own affects
in order to confirm and bestow upon the inner experience a certain
perceptual validity. It would appear that the growing child requires
the confirmation of the *other* to claim possession of her own affects.

There are many patients who require that their therapist identify
what they are feeling because they lack the capacity to perceive their
own affects. Although they are not aware of what they are feeling,
something is communicated to the analyst, not by means of words but
as a metacommunication. The therapist must rely on his own countertransference as a perceptual instrument to identify those affects
that are present in the patient. Such patients do not know about their
love or hatred of the analyst; they do not know that they are anxious
or depressed. In order to use his own countertransference as a perceptual instrument, the analyst must first recognize his collusion in the
patient's emotional *absence*.

Prototypical deficiencies in affective experience include the following: (1) failures in the process of containment of affects (implicit here
is that painful or noxious affects are equated with the [bad] self, so
that acceptance of these affects is equated with acceptance of the self);
(2) failures in the process of recognizing and identifying affects (failures in *affect attunement* or empathy); (3) states of psychic deadness
and inauthenticity, in which the therapist is enlisted in providing a
sense of aliveness. In this affective retraining the therapist provides
certain functions that normally would have been internalized. The
extent to which a developmental deficiency can be corrected in later

life can only be answered in each particular case. Although we cannot fully restore what has been missing in development, there is also no doubt that this kind of affective interaction can, for some individuals, be ameliorative.

I am, of course, describing a *corrective emotional experience*. This much-maligned term is associated with Alexander's proposal that the analyst should assume a certain role to differentiate himself from the behavior or personal traits of the patient's parents.[7] Alexander's technical recommendation that the analyst should deliberately behave in a manner that offers a contrast to the patient's caretakers has been justly criticized as a false and condescending manipulation that undermines the patient's autonomy. I have tried to demonstrate that the therapist's affective interactions primarily represent a response to the patient and not the reverse: it is the patient who initiates the affective chain of responses. Furthermore, this process occurs without the introduction of any active measures, that is to say, it occurs within the frame of the therapeutic setting. The therapist's capacity to contain and accept his patient's affects is no doubt facilitated by the asymmetry of the therapist's emotional position vis-à-vis his patient, the asymmetry of desire that I described in Chapter 2.

Some patients who suffer from inauthenticity to such an extent that they feel themselves to be psychically dead may need to evoke the therapist's affects in order to create a sense of psychic aliveness. Such patients need to evoke an affective response in the therapist so that the therapist's affects can be used as a means of "psychic pump-priming" (Modell 1984a). For example, I described a patient who experienced an absence of sexual desire; she attempted to arouse me sexually so that I in turn would "place" some erotic feeling back into her. Other patients will create crises in the treatment or arouse the therapist's response in other ways in order to evoke affects in the therapist that will instill a sense of psychic aliveness in themselves. These affective interchanges recreate affective absences that have occurred in the past; but they occur in a fresh context with the expectation and hope for a second chance.

We can observe that at times patients will use our affective responses as a model to be emulated. Indeed, some affective interchanges with our patients may be unconsciously motivated specifically by this wish to utilize our response as a model to be emulated and internalized. For example, a patient who had great difficulty in tolerating feelings of guilt attempted to make me feel guilty in order to observe how I was able to cope with my guilt. It should be understood, however, that the patient had no conscious awareness that this was his intent. Patients may unconsciously arouse feelings of anger, guilt, or sexual arousal in the therapist in order to provide themselves with a model with which they can identify. This process moves in the opposite direction from Alexander's corrective emotional experience; it is the *patient* who introduces the corrective emotional experiences in order to incorporate the therapist's response.[8]

5

Experiencing Time

In most considerations of the psychology of time, a distinction is made between two different experiences of time: the linear time of the physicists and astronomers—time's arrow in the universe—and cyclic or human time. This distinction corresponds to the Greek terms *chronos,* which refers to sequential and linear time, and *kairos,* which refers to human time, concerned with personal actions and aims (Kairos was the youngest son of Zeus and the God of opportunity). *Kairos* is cyclic time, the mythic time of both repetitive tragedies and new beginnings; it is the time that is celebrated in anniversaries, rituals, and religious ceremonies. *Chronos* is objective, impersonal time that goes ticking on regardless of our aims and intentions; it is the time that is associated with logic and science. Jaques (1982) argues that *chronos* and *kairos* do not refer to different kinds of time but *different modes of organizing experience in time*—that both experiences of time are present simultaneously. We cannot escape our biological clock that informs us of time's arrow, but the organization of our memory system is such that another biological given, events in present time, are given meaning only by evoking memories of the past. Jaques suggests that human beings organize their temporal world along two axes: a dimension of the succession of time, the historical dimension, and the dimension of prediction and intent, which contains the conception of goal-directedness (1982, p. 87).

Eliade (1959) refers to the "myth of the eternal return." He believed that myths, especially religious myths, abolish current or profane time in that an "act becomes real only insofar as it imitates or repeats an archetype. Thus, reality is acquired solely by repetition or participation; everything which lacks an exemplary model is 'meaningless,' i.e. it lacks reality" (1959, p. 34). In religious ceremonies such as acts of sacrifice, the ceremony is performed at the same mythical instant as the original act; here the paradox of time is that *chronos* is present yet abolished. In ritual purification the sins that occurred during the past year are removed; the passage of time seems to be negated with this new beginning. Thus *kairos* and *chronos* coexist, but human experience tends to favor *kairos*.

Because the experience of time itself is fleeting and elusive, discussion of this subject can easily become vague and abstract. Our biological clock is relentless, but the perception of *chronos* is a process that is usually outside of our awareness and does not command our attention. Our attention to the experience of *kairos,* cyclic time, is also usually obscured; we attend to the repetitive ritual and not to the experience of time itself.

Freud is reported by Marie Bonaparte (1940) to have said: "The sense we have in the passing of time originates in our inner perceptions of the passing of our own life. When consciousness awakens in us we perceive this internal flow and project it into the outside world." Thus, the awareness of *chronos* is at bottom *an awareness of the finitude of life and the inevitability of death.* Cyclic time, on the other hand, suggests *timelessness, an escape from the inevitability of death.*

Despite its elusive nature, the experience of time is central to human psychology. Indeed, it has been asserted, with some justification, that the experience of time is the *essence* of human psychology (Jaques 1982). Kafka (1977) also said that mind is time. This was only a rediscovery of what was known to St. Augustine, who observed (397, p. 271): "Time is merely an extension . . . though of what it is an extension I do not know . . . I begin to wonder whether it is an extension of the mind itself." We also owe to St. Augustine the clearest description of the paradox of time:

> For what is time? Who can readily and briefly explain this? . . . If no one asks me, I know: if I wish to explain it to one that asks, I know not: yet I say boldly that I know, that if nothing passed away, time past were not; and if nothing were coming, a time to come were not; and if nothing were, time present were not. Those two times then, past and to come, how are they, seeing the past now is not, and that to come is not yet? (p. 262)

> Whatsoever is . . . is only as present. Although when past facts are related, there are drawn out of the memory, not the things them-

selves which are past, but words which, conceived by the image of the things, they in passing, have through the senses left as traces in the mind. Thus my childhood, which now is not, is in time past, which now is not: but now when I recall its image, and tell of it, I behold it in the present, because it is still in my memory (p. 266) . . . there be three times, past, present, and to come: yet . . . it might be properly said: there be three times: a present of things past, a present of things present, and a present of things future. (p. 265)

T. S. Eliot echoed St. Augustine in the following lines from *Burnt Norton* (1962, p. 117):

> Time present and time past
> Are both perhaps present in time future,
> And time future contained in time past.
>
> What might have been and what has been
> Point to one end, which is always present.

The dynamic interactions between past, present, and future time encompass the different agencies of the mind, the agencies of memory, perception, and desire. From this point of view, as noted in Chapter 1, *the ego is a structure engaged in the processing and reorganizing of time.* Therapeutic change is in essence the reorganization of the experience of time. It can be said that the psychoanalytic and psychotherapeutic settings are designed to maximize and to bring into some juxtaposition the experience of past, present, and future time.[1]

Anna O.'s "chimney sweeping" served to contrast present time with time past. In her collaboration with Breuer, this contrast between present time and the time of the origin of her symptoms became the focus of the curative process. Anna O.'s alternation between her two personalities was an alternation in time between the traumatic year of 1881 and the then current year, 1882. This alternation, which she achieved by means of hypnosis, has its equivalent in contemporary treatment in the experience of the transference; for transference contrasts archaic affective memories of objects with the affects experienced toward the *current* object relationship with the therapist. In the dependent/containing transference, early (maternal) stages of development are reexperienced symbolically by means of the therapist's mimetic actions, while at the same time the therapist is perceived as someone in the here and now. In the other transference mode, that of the iconic/projective transference, there is a reactivation, a repetition of specific affect categories, so that a template of memories of the past is reactivated in current time. In both modes the analyst or therapist becomes an unwitting collaborator in the recreation of the past, while still retaining a proximity to present time. The therapist becomes the person with whom one can reexperience trauma within a new context or experience for the first time what has been absent in the past. Affects belonging to the past that were never expressed then can now be recontextualized in current time. This is not just a simple catharsis but an actual reorganization of memory. It is the process that provides a second chance.

Loewald has asserted that "psychic structures are temporal in nature" (1980, p. 430). He elaborated his position as follows (pp. 44, 45):

> What we call the psychic past, as in transference phenomena, is not "in the past" but in the present; it is active now, yet active as psychic past, it is the actuality of past experiences. The same is true for unconscious memory traces and their relationship to day residues. Both here and in clinical transference phenomena, the psychic past acts on . . . the psychic . . . objective present. But the psychic present also has an impact on the psychic past; it activates the psychic past. Memory, as recollection for instance, manifests psychic time as activity; it makes the past present . . . The remarkable fact is that in mental life the past, that is psychic past, is not in the (objective) past but is active now as past and that the psychic present acts on the psychic past.

In this connection it is of interest to turn again to Freud's letter to Fliess of December 6, 1896, reproduced in the section on *Nachträglichkeit* in Chapter 1. In this letter Freud notes that pathology ensues when the translation of psychic material between successive registrations does not take place, that is, when the experience of the past remains unassimilated and unmodified in present time. If one fully grasps this idea, Freud is stating that it is not the trauma itself that is pathogenic but how that trauma is processed retroactively. If one carries this idea further, one recognizes *a false polarity between the traumatic versus the intrapsychic origin of the neuroses.*

Psychic Trauma and the Domination of Time Past

If the ego (and its substructures) can be thought of as an organ that reorganizes our experience of time, we would also anticipate that in pathological states there will be a disturbance in the dynamic relationship between the experience of past, present, and future time. The retranscription of memory that Freud described has not taken place.

Schiffer (1978) described the effect of a massive psychic trauma in a woman who, during her adolescence, had been an inmate of Nazi prison camps. For her, "the past was experienced as the present; the nightmare of the past became the only prospect for the future" (1978, p. 48). Schiffer described her experience of time as the "telescoping" of the past into the future, with the obliteration of present time.

We also know that the effect of massive trauma of this sort can be passed on to the next generation by means of a form of cultural inheritance. Children of the survivors of the Holocaust will not uncommonly incorporate their parent's experiences as if such events were part of their own past; the parent's memories are assumed by the children and can dominate their experience of present time. A patient reported a feeling of guilt following this seemingly innocuous interaction. In referring to a telephone number, the person at the other end of a phone line said: "I didn't get the [number] four." This comment triggered an inexplicable feeling of guilt, which my patient was able to trace to memories of his father's past that he had assimilated as his own. His father had survived the Holocaust by constructing an underground bunker within the ghetto that he could share with only a limited number of people. Although the father did not express *his* guilt concerning the life-and-death decisions he implicitly made in excluding others, the patient experienced the father's unexpressed guilt and internalized it as if it were his own. The phrase "I didn't get the four" evoked the "memory" of those not rescued and doomed to die. Thus his parent's history was inseparable from his own; and time past (his parent's time past) was transposed into the patient's present time.

Added to the unassimilated memories of earlier trauma of the individual are the memories of the nuclear family. This process is not unlike the collective memories or collective myths of the tribe, which color the experience of present time. In this fashion we all include cultural memories, whether actual or mythical, associated with our race, our religion, our nationality, and so forth. We know that people willingly sacrifice their lives for such "memories." In this age of worldwide rampant nationalism, no one can doubt the impact of the trauma of the past upon the experience of present time.

Freud attributed these borrowed cultural memories to the "ideology" of the superego (1933, p. 67): "Mankind never lives entirely in the present. The past, the traditions of the race and of the people, lives on in the ideologies of the super-ego, and yields only slowly to the influences of the present and to new changes; and so long as it operates through the super-ego it plays a powerful part in human life, independently of economic conditions."

The Manic Defense: The Everlasting Present

In cases of trauma, where the memory of the past is kept alive and is not assimilated, the past dominates and truncates present time; the past can be said to obliterate time. Future time is anticipated to be no more than a repetition of the past. The manic defense presents us with the opposite state of affairs, in that present time is expanded at the expense of the past and the future.[2]

The manic defense was first observed in manic-depressive illness, but it is not confined to individuals liable to develop mania. Winnicott (1958) understood the manic defense as an inability to give full significance to inner, that is, psychic, reality. Painful memories, especially the memory of loss, are denied; it is as if the individual is effectively cut off from memories of the past and concerns about the future. He is in a world of the *everlasting present*. Normally the meanings and significations of current experience are mediated through affective memories of the past, and it is this dimension that is missing. The use of this manic defense can be observed in the treatment setting when patients, for considerable periods, focus exclusively on current events without forming connections between these events and memories of the past. For example, the retelling of episodes within a bad marriage can obliterate everything else.

As Winnicott (1958) described the manic defense, it is a flight from internal reality. Current events are described in abundant and superfluous detail; there is an emphasis on the "thingness" of things, shorn of their affective associations. The manic defense may represent a transient defense in someone who at other times maintains contact with her inner life, or it may represent a central and integral aspect of character. The absence of the experience of *kairos* contributes to the impression that such people are lacking a certain depth or psychological-mindedness. For these individuals the experience of time is not cyclic; it is the one dimension of the everlasting present. In an everlasting present, there is no loss and no death.

The Experience of Timelessness

The denial of *chronos* may be accomplished by other means. The manic defense creates the illusion of the everlasting present in that the experience of present time is not recontextualized with the past. The illusion of timelessness reflects a different structure and a different origin; it may arise from a sense of merger with the protective mother, which recreates a wished-for union with the mother that is outside of time.

Arlow (1984) reported the case of a violinist who, during a concert, experienced a mystical sense of timelessness. The analysis demonstrated that behind this young woman's experience of timelessness there was a pervasive death anxiety as well as a fantasy of merging with the Virgin Mary. The suspension of time, placing oneself outside of time, is evidently a means of negating the dangers of the real world—the inevitability of aging, illness, and death. But I suspect that the suspension of time represents something in addition to an escape from death anxiety, which in any case should not be underestimated. I believe, as Arlow's patient illustrates, that there is also an evocation, as in other mystical experiences such as the "oceanic experience," of a joyful primitive fusion with the protective mother.[3] The experience of timelessness is, as many have noted, related to the *déjà vu* phenomenon, which can also be understood as a defense against death anxiety (Orgel 1965; Arlow 1959).[4]

Other dynamic shifts in the experiencing of time include the experience of nostalgia. This word originally denoted a melancholy homesickness, but the term has undergone a change of meaning and now denotes the preoccupation with pleasurable or at least bittersweet memories of the past (Werman 1977). Perhaps we owe this change of definition to Marcel Proust, whose literary method was such that present time opened up an entire panorama of past experience. One thinks, of course, of his famous recreation in memory of the childhood world of Combray evoked by dipping a morsel of cake in the cup of tea that his mother had presented to him. He said that this former world opened up like Japanese paper flowers unfolding in water. It was suggested (by M. L. Miller) that Proust's work was the crystallization of his nostalgia that "by tapping the well-springs of the past, renewing joys stored in the 'unconscious,' enables Proust to live the true essences of life outside of time—death is overcome by escaping from time" (cited in Werman 1977, p. 394).[5]

The paradox of timelessness has also been presented visually in the work of the Italian painter Giorgio de Chirico, who has been described as the first artist to paint thought. The inner landscape is represented by empty streets and empty buildings, by statues in human form that do not move. The frozen memories of mythic figures are eternally present, but the wind is seen to be in constant motion, reminding the viewer of the existence of *chronos*. As Calvino commented on these works of de Chirico (1986a, p. 88): "Time will no longer have a hold on you, the hourglass remains suspended. All that counts is the memory, which is already present in the present, the uncertainty of the moment that remains changeless and is repeated." Yet in these paintings there is also movement: a fluttering of banners, clouds moving in the sky, and often, in the distance, a ship with its sails catching the wind or a locomotive emitting smoke.

Freud on Time and the Timelessness of the Unconscious

Freud's aphoristic statement that the unconscious is timeless might lead one to conclude mistakenly that Freud was considering the *experience* of timelessness. But what Freud had in mind was something quite different. In Freud's metapsychology, *nothing* is experienced in the unconscious. "Timeless" in this context refers to the timelessness of memories under repression in the unconscious as a system. Freud believed that in the unconscious mind nothing was ever lost; that wishes remained always potentially active (1900, p. 577); that the unconscious was the repository of permanent memory traces, memories separated from the signification that memories acquire through verbal associations. Freud's aphorism that the unconscious is timeless, if it has any meaning at all, refers to a belief that a portion of the mind remains outside of all experience and is therefore also sequestered from time itself. The timelessness of the unconscious is the *absence of experience*. Freud would later state in his paper "The Unconscious" (1915a, p. 187): "The processes of the system Ucs. are *timeless;* i.e. they are not ordered temporally, are not altered by the passage of time; they have no reference to time at all. Reference to time is bound up, once again, with the work of the system Cs."

This conception can be traced to the quasi-neurological "Project for a Scientific Psychology" and does not seem to be at all congruent with Freud's own clinical experience. For in his "Studies in Hysteria," Freud emphasized that it is *affects* that invest memory with signification. Yet in this description of the timelessness of the repressed memories of the unconscious, he does not mention affects and suggests further that these memories are devoid of "sensory qualities" until such memories are joined with consciousness (1900, pp. 540–541). Ricoeur's reading of Freud (1970, p. 148) agrees with my interpretation: that for Freud the unconscious "bears the mark of non-meaning." Freud's assertion that memory is unalterable in the unconscious appears also to be at variance with his concept of *Nachträglichkeit;* but then he allows for the process of retranscription by indicating that memory traces are permanent, but so are the subsequent retranscriptions of those memories (1901, p. 274 n.2):

> In the case of *repressed* memory-traces it can be demonstrated that they undergo no alteration even in the course of the longest period of time. The unconscious is quite timeless. The most important as well as the strangest characteristic of psychical fixation is that all impressions are preserved, not only in the same form in which they were first received, but also in *all the forms which they have adopted in their further developments* [my emphasis].

Freud believed that the *experience* of time requires the participation of the perceptual apparatus; hence the awareness of time is linked to objective or external reality. In his paper "The Mystic Writing-Pad" (1925a, p. 231) Freud envisioned that the system unconscious periodically sends out feelers or bursts of energy that innervate the system Pcpt.-Cs.: "this discontinuous method of functioning of the system Pcpt.-Cs. lies at the bottom of the origin of the concept of time."

If in Freud's metapsychology the system unconscious is devoid of experience, there is, by definition, no empirical means of testing his assertion that the unconscious is timeless; it appears to be a tautology. On the other hand, it may be argued that dreaming supplies some confirmation that the unconscious is timeless. The experiences of childhood are recreated in dreams, and the dead appear as if they are alive. One could argue that in dreaming there is no notice of time's arrow. In such dreams time appears to be suspended, as if nothing that we have ever experienced has been lost. But there are dreams that also testify to an awareness of the passage of time, as well as an awareness of the future.[6] And we know that any experience we have while awake is capable of finding its representation in a dream, and such representations include the experience of linear time.

I would prefer to think of the storage of memories under repression, what Freud thought to be a repository of memory traces outside of time in the system unconscious, as the storage of a *potential* for the evocation of affect categories. Memories have the potential to be reactivated by events in present time. There is no question that memories of the past and current mental processes act synergistically; recall that the compulsion to recreate the affects of a painful experience was in the service of a perceptual process. Edelman (1987) views memory as a form of recategorization based on current input, as something that is "transformational rather than replicative." As described in the previous chapter, Edelman's theory reinforces the view that transference repetition can be thought of as the refinding of affect categories. We know that repetitive transference affects act synergistically with the perceptual system in the process of testing the human environment. Affective memories of the past can only be experienced through the activation of the perceptual system. This activation corresponds to the experience of human or cyclic time, the interpenetration of the past in the present, of which transference is one example. In this sense there is also a biological backing for the experience of cyclic time in addition to the familiar biological clock that informs organisms of the passage of linear time.

Apart from Freud's belief in permanent memory traces, his view of memory and the experience of time was also *transformational*. Freud's view was that the unconscious contained repressed memories, originally derived from experience, but stored outside of experience and remaining without signification until they are brought into some relation to the perceptual system. Edelman said essentially the same thing: memory requires current input for its recategorization. Wollheim (1984) was also describing the same process when he stated (1984, p. 98): "The way in which an earlier event is kept causally alive is through the phenomenology of a later mental state" (p. 98).

Contemporary neurophysiology confirms what Freud knew from his earliest clinical observations—that memories can have experiential immediacy only if they are memories of *affective* experiences. Rosenfeld (1988, p. 164) reports on the work of Pierre Gloor and his colleagues, who investigated memory by means of artificial electrical stimulation of the cortex in patients with epilepsy. They concluded that "unless limbic structures are activated experiential phenomena do not occur." They state further: "Attaching some affective or motivational significance to a percept may be the specific limbic contribution to this process. This may be the precondition for the percept to be consciously experienced or recalled and may imply that all consciously perceived events must assume some kind of affective dimension, if only ever so slight."

Narration and Human Time

Ricoeur said in his book *Time and Narrative* (1984, p. 52) that "time becomes human to the extent that it is articulated through a narrative mode, and narrative attains its full meaning when it becomes a condition of temporal existence." The pleasure in narrative, Ricoeur suggests, is *the pleasure obtained from the reconfiguration of time*. This pleasure can be multiplied, as in the *Odyssey,* where one finds narratives nested within narratives. The adventures of Odysseus are interrupted by the narration of the actions of the Gods in present time, and the narrative action of Odysseus's adventures is interrupted by the song of the blind minstrel harper, who describes the lives of the Gods in time past.

There has been considerable interest in narration as a fundamental mode of explanation in psychoanalysis. For example, Roy Schafer takes the radical position that nearly everything in the psychoanalytic encounter is narrative. In his book *The Analytic Attitude* (1983, p. ix) Schafer says: "I focus on the presupposition [that] . . . the structure and logical justification of interpretation . . . is a form of narration through *creating* life histories and treatment histories" (my emphasis). The analysand's case history is a narrative,[7] as are also the analysand's resistance and defense. Even psychoanalytic theory is seen as narrative; Schafer suggests that Freud's instinct theory can be thought of as a story of "the young child as a beast." Schafer's assertion that the narrative mode is fundamental to psychoanalysis is shared by Spence (1982), who has also emphasized that the analyst's interpretation is not veridical since the historical truth of an individual's life cannot be known; it is not a question of truth but a matter of "narrative fit." These authors find support for their position in that the narrative mode is considered by some as an alternative way of ordering experience, of constructing reality. It is an alternative to what Bruner (1986) calls the *logico-scientific mode*—an alternative to the scientific quest for truth. The narrative mode addresses the question of how we endow experience with meaning.

Whatever the philosophical status of the narrative mode may be, when it is applied to psychoanalysis there seems to be a confusion between literature and the investigation of human psychology. Even if we put aside for the moment the controversy concerning the "placement" of psychoanalysis, whether it is a scientific or a hermeneutic discipline,[8] the fact remains that human lives are not an open narrative whose story lines can be capriciously altered in one direction or another. The analogy between psychoanalysis and the narrative text has been overextended and ultimately cannot be supported because it ignores the fundamental fact that I have been emphasizing in this book: *the past cannot simply be reconstructed arbitrarily because it is rooted in ineradicable affective experiences.* Affects are a biological phenomenon essential to our survival, and as such, they are central in social evolution, as Freud well understood. It is affects that provide meaning and significance to our past; as I noted in an earlier publication (Modell 1984), affects are at the crossroads of biology and history. While it is true that a narrative reconfigures time, the narrative mode when applied to an actual life can only reconfigure time within the constraints of specified affective memories. The narrative mode in psychoanalysis, unlike that of literature, has biological constraints.

Although the narrative mode provides a sense of intelligibility and coherence, the search for coherence is not always a deeply felt human need except for those few individuals who cherish understanding. On the face of it, the invocation of the narrative mode appears to be a hermeneutic alternative to Freud's grounding of psychoanalysis in an evolutionary biology. But then one must ask: what deep human need is gratified by the act of narration? Narration does not sustain any vital order of human existence, such as self-preservation, sexuality, or aggression. Narration does, however, reinforce the dimension of *kairos,* the experience of human time.

Man assumes that he alone has an awareness of death, but this may not be true. The more we discover about animal intelligence, the less secure we are in our belief in our own unique abilities (Hearne 1986). Wollheim also questions the definition of a person in terms of the experience of time (1984, p. 31): "A person leads his life at a crossroads: at the point where a past that has affected him and a future that lies open meet in the present. But this, if true of the person, is true of every other thing, animate creature and inanimate object." Nevertheless, it does seem probable that only human beings have an awareness of their own history, and that only human beings are influenced by an imaginative reconstruction of the past, a past that includes not only memories but also fantasies. From this one can conclude that the full experience of *kairos,* human time, may be synonymous with insight or the examined life.

6

The Act of Interpretation

Interpretation enjoys a very special status in psychoanalysis. Making an interpretation has been viewed as the pinnacle of an imagined hierarchy of therapeutic procedures that include suggestion, manipulation, and clarification (Bibring 1954). As Freud learned to his misfortune in the case of Dora,[1] to neglect the interpretation of the transference will imperil the treatment itself. Although the need for a transference interpretation at certain critical points in the treatment is unquestioned, it is not entirely clear how making an interpretation preserves the treatment. The act of interpretation cannot be reduced to the simple formula "making the unconscious conscious" because it is a complex interaction between two people, a transactional event. I am therefore in agreement with Klauber (1981, p. 31), who said: "It seems to me that one of the difficulties in the theory of the therapeutic process has been the tendency to see too much from the point of view of the content of interpretation at the expense of adequate study of the meaning of interpretation in the complex relationship of mutual transference."

We must recognize that the act of interpretation is one of great complexity, and it may not always be possible to separate the mimetic or symbolic meaning of making an interpretation from the therapeutic effect of the ostensive content, of the words themselves. A patient may respond primarily to the metacommunication rather than to the content of an interpretation. This observation has long been recognized: interpretations may be experienced as a feeding (good or bad), as a phallic penetration, as a gift from the analyst, and so forth.

There are some patients who are so cut off from their affective life that transference interpretations are impossible. Yet it is clear that these patients can achieve significant therapeutic benefit from the analyst's mimetic actions, such as those that contribute to the illusion that the analytic setting is a holding environment. As a consequence, early developmental conflicts can be actualized. Although the therapeutic benefits may not be definitive, the gains that are achieved cannot be dismissed as the result of reassurance or as the result of active, supportive measures, because such measures have played no part in the curative process. I described earlier how the psychoanalytic setting is the medium through which the process of symbolic actualization occurs, a process in which it is possible through the analyst's mimetic action to symbolize and bring into some juxtaposition the patient's experiences with archaic objects and with the new and current relationship to the analyst. In this sense mimesis accomplishes something that is analogous and perhaps equivalent to the act of interpretation; for we know that mimetic actions without ostensive verbal content have profound therapeutic effects.

But the act of interpretation, unlike such symbolic actualizations or enactments, is mediated through verbal langauge. Viderman (1979) makes the point that whether or not the unconscious is structured as a language, as Lacan has asserted, it is by means of language that the unconscious becomes conscious. The psychoanalytic interpretation has its ground in the verbal *dialogue* between the two participants; the interaction is mediated through language. Interpretation can be realized only through the interchange of meanings between the persons involved (Leavy 1973, 1980). But mimesis can also create meaning; for example, the therapist who accepts a gift from a patient who believes that the inside of his body is bad and dangerous is, through the acceptance of the gift, communicating something that is equivalent to the interpretation: "In valuing your gift I acknowledge that what is inside you is good." Thus we are left to consider the following questions: Are the analyst's actions experienced symbolically, inferior to verbal interpretations? When can such actions function as an equivalent to an interpretation and when can they not?

Language, unlike symbolic enactments, is a reflection of each individual's constructed world; every person has a private store of meanings, a private symbolic treasury (Leavy 1973). An interpretation, unlike a piece of mimetic action, exposes, through language, this private world. Laplanche and Pontalis (1973, p. 227) defined an interpretation as "a procedure which, by means of analytic investigation, brings out the latent meaning in what the subject says or does." But this definition does not address the question: does the interpretation represent the analyst's meaning or the patient's meaning? To what extent is the interpretation the analyst's creation and to what extent does it correspond to the contents of the patient's mind? The act of interpretation, therefore, confronts us with the additional problem: whose reality is it?

The making of an interpretation is a transactional act that cannot be separated from the state of relatedness between the analyst and the patient at the precise moment the interpretation is given. This state of relatedness will determine whether the interpretation represents a shared reality, a shared creativity, or whether it represents predominantly the analyst's reality. The act of interpretation, which uncovers hidden meanings, in itself creates additional meanings.

The Therapeutic Action of Transference Interpretations

The single most influential paper on the theory of treatment, other than Freud's papers on psychoanalytic technique, has been James Strachey's "The Nature of the Therapeutic Action of Psychoanalysis" (1934). Much of the recurrent discussion concerning the therapeutic effects of transference interpretation has been a gloss on Strachey's thesis: that the fulcrum of therapeutic action in psychoanalysis is the "giving"[2] of transference interpretations *at the point of [affective] urgency*. Strachey's point of urgency is equivalent to what I have described earlier as the activation, within the transference, of affect categories. "Making" an interpretation at the point of affective urgency creates a contrast between archaic affect categories and those experienced in the here and now in relation to the analyst. Strachey gave as an example a patient who, in the transference, is experiencing archaic aggressive affects toward the analyst. If the interpretation is successful, such a patient will experience the *contrast* between his archaic object and the real nature of the analyst. The analyst, in the process of making an interpretation, will disconfirm the patient's archaic image or fantasy of the object or of the self. The essential point is that the analyst, in the act of making an interpretation, at the point of affective urgency, *is simultaneously reestablishing the borders between different levels of reality and retranscribing past time in the context of a new and current reality.* Archaic affect categories are recontextualized through the action of the analyst as a current and "real" object.

Fenichel (quoted in Panel 1937) reaffirmed Strachey's theory when he said: "The prime essential of a transference interpretation in my view is that the feeling or impulse interpreted should not be merely concerned with the analyst but that it should be *in activity* at the moment at which it is interpreted." (my emphasis). This is in effect a "procedure which enables the patient to employ his sense of reality for the purpose of making a comparison between his archaic imaginary objects and his actual and real ones."

When transference and countertransference interactions take the form of a projective identification, the interpretation of the transference is obligatory; it is in effect an emergency measure needed to preserve the treatment. As I described earlier, during the process of projective identification there is a commingling of the patient's and the therapist's inner reality that results in a sense of confusion for both participants. This confusion reflects the loss of the apperception (on the part of both participants) of distinct and separate levels of reality within the treatment setup. This represents, in effect, a rupture of the frame of the treatment: the analyst falls out of the frame. Ultimately, it is only by means of transference interpretations that the rupture can be repaired. Projective identification is, to be sure, an extreme instance, but it throws into bold relief a process that is probably always present in those transference/countertransference experiences where intense affects are communicated.

Freud at one point made the analogy that the unconscious of the analyst and the unconscious of the patient were connected like the microphone of a telephone and its receiver (Freud 1912a, p. 115). When transference affects with their associated fantasies are transmitted in this fashion to the analyst, she in turn, must be able to distinguish whether the affect category originated within the patient or within herself, for the communication of intense affects necessarily evokes a complementary response. For example, a patient who consistently belittles and attacks the analyst and her technique may, if the analyst is inclined to be self-critical, evoke in the analyst a sense of defectiveness. The analyst must be clear that in this particular instance she is perceiving something that has its origin in the patient. When the analyst has accomplished this task of separating within her own mind these different levels of reality, she is then able, by means of the act of interpretation, to facilitate a similar process in the patient's mind. As Klauber observed (1981), it is not only the patient who may be relieved by the act of interpretation; it may be a regulator of psychic tension for the analyst as well.

The act of interpreting, in addition to reestablishing the separateness of levels of reality, facilitates the reconfiguration of time. Thus the interpretation of the transference promotes the full experience of human or psychic time. When Freud described (in his letter to Fliess of December 6, 1896) his theory of memory as a retranscription, he also suggested that when this process is impeded, psychopathology ensues: ". . . [a] translation that has not taken place in the case of some of the material which has certain consequences." Psychopathology occurs when certain memories are sequestered from the modifying influence of subsequent experience; it is another way of stating that "hysterics suffer from reminiscences." The tyranny of the past loosens its hold upon us when there are successive retranscriptions of memory. This is precisely what is accomplished by means of transference interpretations, given at the point of affective urgency; transference interpretations facilitate the experience of *kairos,* cyclic time. The retranscription by means of transference interpretation is analogous to the work of mourning in that the effect is cumulative, the result of innumerable small steps.

The Specificity of Transference Interpretations

Does the content of an interpretation matter? Or is the act of interpretation sufficient in itself to achieve a therapeutic effect? Does it matter what the analyst says to the patient, or is it simply enough for the analyst, through the act of interpretation, to reestablish his role within the frame? Is the content of the interpretation always the analyst's construction, or can it be a true observation?

Some analysts, such as Schafer (1983) and Spence (1982), have proposed a theory of interpretation that says in effect that the content of an interpretation is always the analyst's construction and as such is arbitrary. Schafer and Spence believe that interpretations cannot be reconstructions of the past because the past can never be truly known; thus interpretations can only be the analyst's constructions. Of course interpretations are always filtered through the mind of the analyst and therefore undergo a certain transformation, but Schafer and Spence do not acknowledge the special position of transference interpretations in which the analyst's interpretations arise directly from the perception of the patient's state of affective urgency which is directed toward the analyst. Psychoanalytic interpretations, according to these authors, are seen as no different from the interpretation of a text: they both speak of the interpretation as achieving a certain "narrative fit." Schafer calls it the "analyst's story lines," and Spence asserts that interpretations depend more on their power to persuade, on their linguistic characteristics, than on their "truthfulness."

The literary critic Frank Kermode, in a brilliant essay entitled "Freud and Interpretation" (1985), described some recent developments in the history of ideas that support the theory of interpretation proposed by Schafer and Spence. Kermode illustrated how certain assumptions concerning the historical past that were bolstered by the sciences of geology and biology during Freud's lifetime have more recently been modified by the science of linguistics. In linguistics it is more profitable to understand how things are, in all their complexity, than to understand how they got that way. There has been, as Kermode notes, a "flight from history" in the interpretative disciplines.

In accordance with this ahistorical premise of modern linguistics, Schafer believes, a priori, that the analysand "can never have direct access to [past] events" and that his experience of these events is always subjective and therefore open to further, interminable interpretation. The analyst's interpretations are "acts of retelling or narrative revision" (Panel 1983, p. 240). An "accurate" interpretation is an impossibility because the analyst is only offering the patient an alternative "story line"; he is merely substituting *his* narrative for that of the patient.

If memory is a retranscription, if there is no permanent record in the brain that is isomorphic with past events, than all memories are in the nature of reconstructions. But even granting this intrinsic fallibility of memory, it would be foolish to assert that one cannot form any judgment regarding the existence of past events. From our patient's accounts we cannot always distinguish actual events from fantasy, as Freud painfully discovered; but in some though not all instances it is quite possible to separate fact from fantasy. In this endeavor we function not too differently from the members of a jury, who also can, in many instances, establish the truthfulness of events in the past with relative certainty.[3]

It is correct, however, as these critics assert, that interpretations are to some extent always a product of the mind of the interpreter, but when the analyst responds to the analysand's affective communication, the interpretation is not arbitrary. For transference interpretations are built upon the analyst's perception of a specific affective experience. There is, then, an important distinction to be made between mutative transference intepretations, as described by Strachey, and interpretations that are made at times of relative (affective) quietude, when there is an absence of affective urgency. Such interpretations have been called *extratransference interpretations*. This term is somewhat misleading because such interpretations may also be references to the transference in the absence of affective urgency. From this we may infer that the greater the affective intensity (directed toward the analyst), the more likely it is that an interpretation will reflect the contents of the analysand's rather than the analyst's mind. (This statement assumes that the analyst has the capacity to receive the patient's communication and to distinguish his or her own affective reactions from those of the patient. In other words, I am assuming a "good enough" analyst.)

When the analyst is not experiencing the patient's transference affects directly, extratransference interpretations are more in the nature of the analyst's constructions: they may represent, as Schafer says, the analyst's "story line." In constrast, transference interpretations reflect the analyst's perceptions of an affect-laden memory (or fantasy) that is saturated with specific mental content. The analyst, in reflecting these perceptions back to the patient, will of course modify and select what is communicated to the patient: but if the analyst's receiver is open and functioning as it should, it is the patient's transmissions that are received.

Schafer's theory of interpretation is in marked contrast to the position taken in 1931 by Edward Glover in his paper "The Therapeutic Effect of Inexact Interpretation." Glover believed that the precise content of an interpretation was of great significance in that an incomplete or inaccurate interpretation would function as the analyst's suggestion and reinforce the patient's defenses (1931, p. 559): "Unless we analyze the content of the mind and uncover the mental mechanisms dealing with this content together with its appropriate affect, we automatically range ourselves on the side of mental defense." According to Glover, the content of a fantasy must be uncovered with precision. Anything less, any inexact interpretation, would introduce elements of the *analyst's mind,* a form of suggestion. Although hardly any analyst today would share Glover's almost puritanical fervor for the need for completeness and accuracy of interpretation, his paper leads to the heart of the problem that I have been considering: does the content of an interpretation represent that which exists within the patient's mind, or is it a creation of the analyst's mind?

The issue of "whose reality is it" is not an abstract philosophical question; indeed, for some patients it may be a very lively concern. Recent developments in cognitive science (Bruner 1986) as well as neurobiology (Edelman 1987) support Piaget's position that every person's perceptual system is unique: perception of reality is always a personal *construction*. Piaget's psychology forms an empirical base for what has become a "constructivist" philosophy.[4] Nelson Goodman, a notable proponent of this point of view, states (1984, p. 14): "I am convinced that there is no one correct way of describing or picturing or perceiving '*the world*,' but rather that there are many equally right but conflicting ways—and thus, in effect, many actual worlds." This philosophical position is consistent with Edelman's observation (1987) that there is a great range of individual variation in the development of the central nervous system: it is not as genetically hard-wired as had been previously supposed. As a result, each individual essentially constructs his or her own view of reality. Modern science has confirmed what William Blake apprehended intuitively: "A fool sees not the same tree that a wise man sees." Thus the analyst, responding with an interpretation to the analysand's point of affective urgency, is perforce constructing his own view of that particular piece of reality, but the construction is based on information received from the patient so that the interpretation is not an arbitrarily constructed "story line."

Learning from the Therapist's Experience

There is an evident dilemma in learning: the child constructs his own view of reality but at the same time is totally dependent on his caretaker's construction of reality for his safety in the world. That is, the child's constructed reality does not assure his survival in the real world. For the infant and the young child, it is the mother who creates an alternative environment that is interposed between the child and the dangers of the external world. In a certain sense the mother *is* reality in that she is the source of vital information concerning the world. For the infant and young child this information is communicated affectively through the mother's face, especially her eyes, her tone of voice, and her entire expressive musculature. With the acquisition of language the child is then dependent upon the parent's judgment, which can for some parents reflect an eccentric and quite idiosyncratic world view. Not infrequently, intelligent children correctly judge that their parent's view of reality is "off," which may have profound consequences for the child's further development. These children learn that their world view is apt to be more dependable and reliable than that of their parents; as a result, they tend not to learn from others in the sense of truly incorporating knowledge and making it their own. Learning for these children is compliant and, in Winnicott's sense, becomes a feature of the false self. They trust only what they learn for themselves.[5] Such individuals, if they enter psychoanalysis, may act as if they are learning from the analysis, but the analyst discovers that he has been writing in sand, that nothing has been truly assimilated. For these patients, to really take in the analyst's interpretation would threaten the continued existence of their self-constructed world.

As Bruner observes (1985), there is a deep parallel in all forms of knowledge acquisition in that the assimilation of knowledge requires a crucial match between a *support system* and an *acquisition process* in the learner. Psychoanalysis as well as other psychologies have paid special attention to the process of internalization, which is the aim of all successful learning and the hoped-for result of interpretation. But psychoanalysis, in contrast to the psychologies of Piaget and Vygotsky, has not paid sufficient attention to the phase of learning that occurs before internalization has taken place. One possible exception to this statement is Winnicott's theory of potential space, a space of shared realities that can be said to belong to neither the subject nor the object.

Vygotsky and Learning from Others

Vygotsky was a Russian psychologist, considered by many to be Piaget's equal, who died in 1934 and whose work is only now beginning to have an impact in the West. Vygotsky's stature can be attested by the fact that Bruner (1985, p. 145) compares Piaget, Vygotsky, and Freud by stating that each one represents a different cultural posture: "Freud faces the present from the past: growth is by freeing. Piaget respects the inviolate integrity of the present: growth is the nurturing of intrinsic logic. And Vygotsky turns the cultural past into the generative present by which we reach toward the future: growth is reaching."

Piaget's theory of learning is primarily a theory of the child's construction of reality—learning that is the result of self-acquired experience, with the role of the teacher omitted. For this reason Piaget's intrapsychic theory of learning was considered by Vygotsky to be solipsistic (Vygotsky 1986). For Vygotsky, learning is interpersonal from the beginning. In contrast to Piaget, Vygotsky examined the process by means of which the child learns from others, that is, the process through which a culture is internalized. Like Winnicott, Vygotsky paid special attention to the facilitating environment.

If we ask the question, whose knowledge is it that is interiorized in a psychoanalysis? there are three possibe answers: learning from one's own experience (within the analysis); learning from the analyst; and the learning that arises spontaneously and cannot be attributed to either patient or analyst because it represents a shared creativity. These three forms of learning have been the province, respectively, of Piaget, Vygotsky, and Winnicott. Winnicott considered this process not under the heading of learning but under that of creativity.

Piaget's theory of assimilation and accommodation describes in essence the dialectic between the child's imposing his own schemata upon the world, that is, creating the world solipsistically, and his subsequent adaptation to an unmoved external reality by means of accommodation. Piaget said (1954, p. 385) that the child subjects "the appearance of things to an egocentric assimilation [and conversely] the assimilation of things to the self is constantly held in check by the resistance necessitating this accommodation, since there is involved at least the appearance of reality, which is not unlimitedly pliant to the subject's will."

Vygotsky investigated a very different question: how does the less competent individual learn from the more competent? His answer was (as described in Bruner 1985, p. 24):

The tutor or the aiding peer serves the learner as a vicarious form of consciousness until such time as the learner is able to master his own action through his own consciousness and control [my emphasis]. When the child achieves that conscious control over a new function or conceptual system, it is then that he is able to use it as a tool. Up to that point the tutor in effect performs the critical function of "scaffolding" the learning task to make it possible for the child, in

Vygotsky's word, to internalize external knowledge and convert it into a tool for external control.

What I find of significance for psychoanalysis here is Vygotsky's description of an intermediate stage of learning before internalization has taken place. Prior to this internalization, the psychoanalyst's knowledge is used vicariously as a tool or as a scaffolding or a "prosthesis." This is analogous to the kind of learning that Vygotsky attributed to the mother: "The child is permitted to do as much as he can spontaneously do: *whatever he cannot do is filled in or "held-up" by the mother's scaffolding activities*" (Bruner 1985, p. 28). In describing the acquisition of language, Vygotsky (1986, p. xxxviii) depicted inner speech as the psychological interface between a private language and culturally sanctioned symbols. We might posit a similar intermediate stage that is an interface between the patient's private world and the acceptance of the analyst's interpretations. For some patients internalization never occurs, and thus they are permanently dependent upon the use of the analyst as a prosthesis.[6] This continued dependency upon the analyst to supply some missing elements of consciousness helps to explain why some analyses are interminable.

Vygotsky is famous for his concept of the *zone of proximal development*, which he describes as follows (quoted in Bruner 1985, p. 24): "the distance between the actual developmental level as determined by independent problem solving and the level of potential development as determined through problem solving under adult guidance or in collaboration with more capable peers." There is much here that resonates with the psychoanalytic situation. The learner, who is in a less developed position, vicariously borrows from the more advanced developmental position of the tutor (the zone of proximal development). In this process, the more advanced teacher acts as a support system that fills in the gaps in those levels of development which the student has not yet acquired.[7]

In psychoanalysis this method of acquiring knowledge from the more advanced teacher is not limited only to the act of interpretation; it also encompasses what has been described as the *analytic attitude* (Schafer 1983). This analytic attitude includes attitudes toward life and living that can be described as an analytic Weltanschauung (world view). A psychoanalytic Weltanschauung includes a certain attitude toward living and the assumption of the virtues of an examined life. More specifically, it includes a search for unconscious meaning behind all thoughts and actions. In this search there is also an ethical position that states that only behaviors and not thoughts have ethical consequences; the psychoanalyst fosters an empathic examination of all experiences while maintaining a moral neutrality or objectivity. This more accepting, reasonable attitude regarding matters of conscience and morality undoubtedly contributed to the therapeutic effect of psychoanalysis in earlier decades, when the psychoanalytic Weltanschauung stood in contrast to some of the conventional, middle-class cultural values. This is what Strachey (1934) observed when he attributed a leading element in the therapeutic action of pyschoanalysis to the function of the analyst as an "auxiliary superego." The analysand vicariously assumes the altered consciousness associated with the analyst's milder and more "objective" superego while retaining alongside it her own archaic superego. Today, when so much of Freud's teachings have become a part of contemporary culture (albeit in an adulterated and bowdlerized version), the ethical position of psychoanalysis is less noticeable. This Weltanschauung includes more than language, as it extends to what has been described as the analyst's emotional position as well. When the analyst demonstrates a level of affective competence that is, one hopes, in advance of that of the analysand, this level of competence serves as a vicarious form of consciousness for the analysand. The analyst is able to assume a more mature emotional position because of the asymmetry of his needs vis-à-vis those of the analysand; this allows the analyst a greater latitude of impulse control and facilitates his capacity to contain the analysand's noxious affects.

The use of the analyst as a scaffolding or prosthesis has been more commonly recognized under the concept of the use of the analyst as an "auxiliary" ego or superego. There is then an intermediate stage or interface, as Vygotsky suggested, between the analysand's constructed reality and the analyst's world view in which the analyst's communications are used as a vicarious form of consciousness. (This can occur despite Freud's disclaimer that psychoanalysis does not possess a Weltanschauung of its own.)[8] In addition to this shared or communal psychoanalytic Weltanschauung, every analyst has his own private construction of psychoanalysis. For this reason it has been said that the analyst's analyst is always a hidden presence; analysts of different schools speak in different dialects.

All patients vicariously borrow from this scaffolding that their therapists provide. However, for some, the analytic attitude is a graft that does not fully take; it does not become a tool in Vygotsky's sense. Such patients require the continued presence of the analyst or therapist to use the analytic tool. There are individuals who remain psychologically "deaf" and can only hear through the analyst's ears.

Winnicott's Potential Space of Shared Realities

The reader will recall that Winnicott's theory of potential space refers to the illusionary space contained within the therapeutic frame, where "playing" can take place. The participants of the "game" are sharing illusions. Winnicott illustrated the use of this potential space in his squiggle game, in which Winnicott makes a squiggle drawing and then the child turns it into something else; then the child makes a squiggle and Winnicott in turn transforms it into something else. The squiggle is an objectified representation, something that had been internal and is now part of the "objective" world and can henceforth be treated as a "thing" by both participants. Within this potential space we do not ask the question: "whose reality is it?" There are times when the analyst's interpretations and the patient's responses are very much like a squiggle game. It is a transactional sharing of the constructed realities of both participants, leading to a *new construction*.

At times dream interpretation can become a squiggle game. The patient's dream, although the product of his mind, becomes an object, a "thing" for both patient and analyst.[9] The patient presents the dream; the analyst then focuses on a particular element of the dream because it evokes an affective and associative response (the analyst has in effect entered into the patient's creation). The patient, in turn, then produces fresh associations, which evoke a further response on the part of the analyst, and so on. The important point here again is that we do not ask, "whose reality is it?" It is the hallmark of a "good" hour when one does not quite know whether it is the patient or the analyst who has made the interpretation.

Interpretation with or without Affects

I have tried to demonstrate that the act of interpretation is not a uniform procedure analogous to those found in medicine. The act of interpretation is a complex transactional process whose meaning will be determined by multiple factors, including the question: whose reality is it? Despite this complexity, it is possible to differentiate the function of affect-laden transference interpretations from extratransference interpretations or transference interpretations without intense affects. For it is only the former that are mutative inasmuch as the presence of specific affect categories are necessary to differentiate current from archaic levels of reality. The reactivation of archaic affects that have invested the self and former objects at the precise moment the interpretation is given enables archaic images of the self and of objects to be differentiated. Extratransference interpretations and interpretations given at points where the affective component is less active serve cognitive and educational functions, for example, the "filling in" of cognitive gaps where the analysand vicariously borrows the analyst's more advanced level of functioning. A theory of treatment requires that we tease out these separate functions of the act of interpretation. For these reasons, Strachey's observation that transmuting interpretations occur only at the point of (affective) urgency, and Fenichel's recognition that feelings toward the analyst should be *in activity* at the precise moment during which the interpretation is made, assume added significance.

7

The Schizoid Dilemma and Other Forms of Resistance

The analysis of resistance, along with the analysis of transference, marked the route that psychoanalysis traveled when it diverged from hypnosis. Freud believed that it was the concept of defense that not only distinguished psychoanalysis from hypnosis but also separated Freudian psychoanalysis from Breuer's theory of psychological treatment (Freud 1923). As a result, resistance has enjoyed a special position as a defining concept in the history of psychoanalysis. Although resistance is, by definition, that which opposes therapeutic change, the arousal of resistance was also seen by Freud as paradoxically positive in that it was a guarantee against the misleading effects of suggestive influence (Freud 1923).

A theory of psychoanalytic treatment seeks to establish certain conceptual tools that will synthesize and unify a wide range of observation. The concept of resistance has proved to be less than an effective tool because the term itself is overly inclusive and lacks precision; for we know that anything that is evoked by the therapeutic process can become a focus of resistance. This is reflected in Freud's classification of resistance, which included the entire psychic apparatus. Freud lists five kinds of resistance (Freud 1926, p. 160): three emanating from the ego, the other two from the id and the superego, respectively. Repression, transference resistance, and the secondary gain of illness arise from the ego. Id (instinctual) resistance is the resistance of repetition, that which requires "working through."[1] Superego resistance is expressed as the sense of guilt and the need for punishment which are in opposition to recovery and the diminution of pain.[2]

Freud's use of the term *resistance* included opposition to the ultimate aims of treatment, that is, resistance to recovery from neurotic suffering, as well as resistance to the therapeutic process itself, such as the resistance to the acceptance of the therapist's interpretation. Clarity is further obscured inasmuch as Freud continued to think of resistance as a quasi-neurological, intrapsychic process ("anticathexis") while at the same time recognizing that, for the most part, resistance took the form of transference resistance, an interpersonal process (Freud 1926, pp. 157–164). The term *resistance* should thus be seen not as a uniform concept but more as an umbrella that covers a very heterogeneous range of phenomena that are grouped together only in their opposition to therapeutic change.

The terms *defense* and *resistance* are nearly indistinguishable, but it has been customary to use *defense* to refer to behavior that is operative in ordinary life, which then becomes a resistance when the individual seeks treatment. Defenses are both intrapsychic and intrapersonal.[3] But since the term *resistance* refers only to the therapeutic process, it is not possible to think of resistance as anything other than an interpersonal process.

How are the forces of resistance overcome? Freud's answer was that the repressing powers (the forces of the anticathexes) could only be overcome through love, that is, through the love of the analyst taken in its broadest context (Freud 1907). If resistance is overcome through love, it is a short step to recognize that resistance is a force directed against an object relationship. The "schizoid" state of non-relatedness can then be understood as a category of resistance.

Despite the fact that the term *resistance* does not lend itself to theorizing, every theory of therapeutic action must of necessity include particular views concerning resistance. If one continues to believe that the aim of treatment is to make the unconscious conscious (an intrapsychic process), resistance is defined accordingly. For example, Rangell (1983) begins his essay on resistance with the categorical statement: "Resistance is a defense against insight." Kohut (1984), on the other hand, condemns the concept of defense and resistance as representative of an antiquated nineteenth-century mechanistic scientism. Schafer (1983) also condemned the concept for its scientism and instead preferred to understand resistance as a narrative. Resistance and defense suggest not only mechanistic metaphors but militaristic ones as well: resistance invariably evokes the military metaphor of force, and defense connotes entrenchment. In keeping with this military analogy, Wilhelm Reich (1949) referred to character defenses as "character armor."

For the reasons just discussed, I will not attempt any systematic view of resistance but will consider the particular forms of resistance that are evoked by various modes of therapeutic action. If one believes that the therapeutic setting together with the affective communication that is facilitated by that setting is the principal motor of change, a defense against relatedness becomes a significant form of resistance. The therapeutic setting has the additional function of *facilitating an environment that is experienced as safe enough to contain multiple and separate levels of reality*. This is an environment that, we hope, will facilitate the experience of *kairos*, cyclic time, so that trauma that truncates present and future time and the manic defense that negates time past and time future can become significant forms of resistance against the experience of cyclic time. In accordance with the theory of treatment that I have outlined, resistance consists of that which interferes with the capacity to apperceive the multiple levels of reality that are present within the psychoanalytic setting. This statement is an extension of what Winnicott said in his condensed, aphoristic style (1971, p. 47): "Psychotherapy has to do with two people playing together . . . where playing is not possible then the work done by the therapist is directed toward bringing the patient from a state of not being able to play into a state of being able to play."

The Schizoid Defense and the Regulation of Closeness

I shall make the assumption that schizoid withdrawal is a defense against relatedness and is ubiquitous (Modell 1975, 1984a). We learn most from extreme instances of character pathology, but we also know that there is no clear line of demarcation between normality and pathology.

The fundamental dilemma of the schizoid person can be stated quite simply: closeness to others threatens the existence and continuity of the self, but withdrawal may lead to a sense of deadness of the self which, if unrelieved, may threaten the individual's attachment to reality. The solution, of course, is to find the proper distance.[4] For the schizoid patient, the privacy of the self is a matter of survival. What the schizoid patient teaches us is that we do not communicate only by means of words; we communicate by means of words charged with a certain quantum of affects. We are all familiar with those patients who fill their hours with talk that communicates nothing, so that at times we feel that we are drowning in a sea of words without meaning. Communication is a regulator of interpersonal distance: affectless communication creates a certain distance between the participants, whereas affect-laden, authentic communication creates a bond between the two participants. Authentic affects are object-seeking; they are that which endows words with meaning.[5] Metacommunication carries information concerning the relationship between the two participants. It is not just the absence of affects that creates distance; false and misleading affects can be used in the service of noncommunication. We are also familiar with patients who create an atmosphere of crisis, of sound and fury that signifies nothing. Thus I must modify my original statement: what endows words with meaning and creates a bond between the participants is a certain quantum of *authentic* affects.

This has been a circuitous way of stating that the schizoid defense against relatedness takes place through the metacommunication of affects. For these patients, the intactness and integrity of their sense of self is threatened by the exposure, sharing, and communication of genuine feeling. It is as if the core of their being is held hostage to the response of the other.

The schizoid defense, which was adaptive in development, later becomes maladaptive and contributes to what we then label as character pathology. These characterological defenses, which are activated by the therapeutic process, will become forces of resistance against recovery. How does this state of affairs come about? I will describe a composite of the patient's answer. This is not intended to be a scientific explanation of the etiology of schizoid states, for we must recognize the existence of a complementary series of genetic determinants acting in concert with environmental determinants. Kagan, Reznick, and Snidman (1988) suggested that a genetically determined hyperactivity of the sympathetic nervous system leads to social inhibition and shyness. A low threshold of interpersonal anxiety will understandably lead to withdrawal. Nevertheless, even though schizoid withdrawal may represent a genetic predisposition in some people, it would be a mistake to believe that this is primarily a biological disorder; for a vulnerability of the sense of self can be traced to a disturbance or a developmental deficiency in the parental holding environment.

I intend to describe certain pathological variations of parent-child interactions which can be recreated symbolically in the interaction between patient and therapist. For some patients, periods of parental overintrusiveness will alternate with other periods of withdrawal and emotional unavailability. One male patient's mother consistently undressed in front of him as if he were not a separate person, as if the sexual differences between them did not really matter. We learned in this instance that the mother did not primarily intend to arouse her son; her exposing herself was more a by-product of her denial that there was any difference between them. Perhaps all acts of intrusion of this sort reveal an insensitivity to the contours and outlines of the child's sense of self and autonomy.

Intrusion can also refer to the bodily self. A female patient's mother did not respect the separateness of her daughter's body in that she successfully toilet trained her by inserting rectal suppositories from the age of six months and thereafter when it was thought to be needed. This same mother insisted that her child adhere to her own quirky dietary convictions, which excluded the ingestion of any sweets; thus the daughter was never permitted to eat candy. This overintrusiveness was paradoxically accompanied by periods in which the mother would be disinterested in the child and would be emotionally absent and unavailable.

These examples of failures in the parental holding environment illustrate the parent's incapacity to respect what can be described as the child's selfhood. Other significant failures of parental holding refer not so much to the parent's inability to accept the child's separateness but to her inability to contain the child's affects, contributing to a fear of annihilation (see Chapter 4). As adults, such patients believe that to share intense feelings risks the annihilation of the self. As one patient put it, she felt as if she were an egg: to share feeling would be to crack herself open, and the precious yolk would run out and be lost forever. The mother's affective response to the child's anxiety may serve either as a faulty or as a protective container. The patient's fear that his therapist will prove to be a faulty container of his affects remains a powerful source of resistance and contributes to the inability of such patients to trust the safety of the therapeutic setting.

Thus the schizoid defense of noncommunication serves multiple needs. Unempathic responses may deplete and shatter the sense of self, as illustrated in the biblical injunction not to cast one's pearls before swine. In addition, the contents of what is inside may be transformed from something wonderful into something bad and destructive when exposed to others, like an apple that spoils when introduced to the air.

Resistance to the Acceptance of the Therapist's Constructed Reality

In the previous chapter I described how the psychoanalyst's Weltanschauung, the analyst's constructed reality, affects the content of an interpretation. Interpretations may be resisted not because the content of the interpretation lifts the barrier of repression but because the interpretation is a representation of the *analyst's* world view. The schizoid patient teaches us that resistance may take the form of a defensive inability to learn from others. For some people, in order to survive it has been necessary to believe implicitly only in their own created reality.

I have also described previously the conflict between the child's created reality and the world view of his caretakers when the child is able to judge that his caretaker's construction of reality is unreliable.[6] For the child is normally dependent upon the parent's judgment of the real world. Not infrequently, intelligent children correctly judge that their parent's view of reality is off. For example, one patient who was in fact intellectually precocious perceived at the age of two or three that his mother was mad, although the extent of her madness was hidden and not acknowledged by her family or neighbors. This child knew that his mother's judgment was unreliable and that she could not assure his safety in the world. Another patient during latency correctly observed his mother to be flighty, childish, and fatuous. This is not to say that the child articulates such observations as I am doing now, but such perceptions are taken in, whether consciously or not, and have profound consequences for the further development of the child. Such a recognition will result in a profound turning away from the caretaker as a source of safety in the world—a rejection of the caretaker's world view. Something analogous, but to a less serious degree, may occur with extremely intelligent children who are brighter than their parents, or children of immigrants who have a greater mastery of the language and local culture than their parents. These children learn that their world view is apt to be more dependable than that of their parents. This loss of their parents as protective objects induces a precocious yet fragile maturation. If this occurs early in development, the child can only sustain himself by relying upon his own constructed reality, at the center of which may be grandiose omnipotent fantasies. For only grandiose omnipotence can make a young child self-sufficient.

The schizoid patient withdraws into a form of "self-holding" which is, in a sense, an alternative world. This loss of the parental holding has profound consequences: in some patients an endopsychic perception is recorded where, as children, they feel themselves to be floating off the world or falling off unsupported into the cold regions of outer space. In later life many schizoid patients report a corresponding endopsychic perception of their self-holding: they feel that they are not really in the world, that they are encased within a plastic bubble, film, bell jar, or, as I have described elsewhere, a "cocoon" (Modell 1984a). One patient reported the feeling that she was encased within a film so that people's faces looked watery. This indefiniteness of people's faces reflected the lack of affective engagement, a detachment from others.

For some patients, this capacity to create an alternative inner world of fantasy may be literally life-preserving. Some degree of self-holding and the creation of alternative self-created worlds must occur in every child, but in the face of significant failures of the holding environment, this caretaker self, which is necessary for survival, becomes hypertrophied. This involves not only a substitution of an internal for an external object but also, in all instances, the creation of an illusion of a separate world; hence the reports by some patients that they are not really "in" the world but are separated from others by an intangible space of unrelatedness.

In such a self-created world one does not communicate to others, nor does one take things in from others. To accept the ideas of another means an acknowledgment of the limits of one's omnipotence; true learning means allowing oneself to enter into someone else's constructed reality. By this means the less experienced person is brought to a higher level of development by the more experienced one, as in Vygotsky's zone of proximal development.

The Therapist's Response to the Patient's Withdrawal

The schizoid patient's state of unrelatedness induces a familiar countertransference response that can also be described as a counter-resistance. In fact, I use this response as a guide to diagnosis. When I am in the continued presence of someone who is not relating to me, I experience a sense of boredom and sleepy withdrawal. Because this response has been reported by others, I am fairly confident that this is not my own peculiarity. Masud Khan, in his introduction to Winnicott's case history of an adult analysis (1986), described this very well as a state of "eerie mellow fatigue." The absence of authentic affects in the patient induces a complementary absence in the therapist. I have observed that some of my students, who are unaware of their own countertransference withdrawal, become inexplicably angry at such patients. To be continuously in the presence of someone who appears to be uninvolved with us is an offense to our narcissistic wish to be responded to.

Winnicott's recently published fragment of an adult analysis was that of a schizoid patient who was, at times, so unrelated that he, the patient, repeatedly fell asleep on the couch. In self-defense, or perhaps to keep awake himself, Winnicott took copious notes, which resulted in this only extensive adult case report. Khan recounts in his introduction to this volume that Winnicott was once asked how one can observe whether someone is truly mentally ill or whether he is basically healthy but only needs some counseling. Winnicott's reply was (1986, p. 1): "If a person comes and talks to you, and listening to him, you feel he is *boring* you, then he is sick and needs psychiatric treatment. But if he sustains your interest, no matter how grave his distress or conflict, then you can help him alright." To recognize this boredom is not a sign of countertransference pique, nor is it calling the patient names. These patients are not necessarily boring as people; it is rather that the boredom is a reflection of the resistance, an interpersonal process of relatedness, an element of which is missing.

I described the schizoid patient as encased in a cocoon where nothing leaves or enters (Modell 1984a). This cocoon can be a veritable fortress. An incapacity to learn from experience is a formidable resistance when it is based on a core of belief within the patient, which has proved to be self-sustaining and life-preserving, that she is at risk if she accepts the therapist's ideas or view of reality. Any ideas that the patient has not already considered herself may be viewed as an alien reality. At bottom, one only accepts the ideas of others if one has abandoned to some degree a belief in personal omniscience. I recall an extreme instance of this problem with a patient whose parents were in fact psychotic and who literally could not accept anything that I said. Even if I paraphrased something that she had just said and in the process introduced something of myself by using my own language, this would provoke a violent rejection. We all have patients who do not hear us. This not hearing serves a multitude of defensive functions, but with schizoid patients it is frequently used to avoid the introduction of alien ideas. Sometimes the not hearing is literal, but mostly it is figurative. Yet we still must figuratively raise our voices in order to be heard, in order to get through. With patients of this sort I find myself unable to use allusion or indirection; at times I must speak bluntly or I will not be heard at all.

This inner world that must not be challenged, threatened, questioned, or otherwise exposed may in some patients assume the dimensions of a private psychosis. I am not thinking of patients who are clinically psychotic; there are many people who are able more or less to maintain themselves in professional and social settings, yet whose inner world is fashioned around fantasies of omnipotence and grandiosity, which if exposed may strike the observer as perfectly crazy ideas. Nevertheless such ideas have proved to be life-preserving in childhood, and for this reason the therapist must approach their exposure with great circumspection. We must also admit that there are some patients whose world view is such that nothing can alter it.

A Paradox of Resistance: The Sphere within the Sphere

When patients are in a state of unrelatedness it is as if they are talking to themselves, but they are talking to themselves in the presence of the therapist. It is, to be sure, a state of non-relatedness, but it is also a state that maintains contiguity with the analyst. I have described this situation with a visual image, that of a sphere within a sphere (Modell 1984a). The sphere of the patient's self-holding, his self-sufficient cocoon, is held within the larger sphere of the psychoanalytic or psychotherapeutic setting. One is reminded here of Winnicott's paper "The Capacity to Be Alone" (1958a). Winnicott viewed the young child's or the infant's capacity to be alone in the presence of the mother as a sophisticated achievement that rests upon a paradox: the capacity to be alone requires the presence of another person. There is a further paradox. States of non-relatedness are states of resistance, since they are essentially states of non-communication. If the aim of the analytic setting is to facilitate free association, states of self-holding withdrawal are certainly in opposition to the basic rule. The paradox is that this state of resistance also facilitates therapeutic change. The therapist both *is* and *is not* a part of the therapeutic process. Healing may be promoted by this state of non-communication and non-relatedness; it is a self-healing that requires the presence of another. Winnicott said (1958a, p. 34): "It is only when alone (that is to say, in the presence of someone) that the infant can discover his own personal life." For the adult patient it is a compromise solution: one in which the resistance of non-communication promotes the process of healing. The therapist must be present but also must be nonintrusive with regard to the patient's self-created world.

There are some patients who are quite comfortable turning their hours into monologues in which the therapist is given no opportunity to say anything other than to make noncommittal noises to acknowledge that she is still there listening. For other patients it is enough to sit in the waiting room as long as the therapist is next door. The sphere of the patient's self-holding, his self-created world, his self-sufficient cocoon, is being held within the larger sphere of the therapeutic setting. Although the patient appears to be talking to himself, to be self-sufficient and unrelated, he is being carried along by the greater sphere of the holding environment provided by the treatment. One must come to trust that this process in fact occurs.

Treatment in this sense proceeds at two separate levels which are split off from each other. Contiguity exists in states of non-relatedness. The patient experiences at a deep level a merging fusion with the therapist, while at the same time being in a state of unrelatedness. In accordance with the induction of a complementary response in the therapist, one can also expect to experience the peculiarity of a sense of merging union at a deep, at times unconscious, level that coexists with a sense of non-relatedness. This is indeed a very peculiar emotional state, for which the therapist may be unprepared because it does not have an analogue in ordinary life.

The Inability to Handle Paradox

Bateson (1972) predicted that certain forms of psychopathology might be characterized by an inability to handle frames and paradoxes; such people would lack the capacity to accept the paradox of the concurrent existence of that which is within the frame and that which is outside. This relative (or absolute) incapacity to use the treatment *creatively* must be acknowledged as another category of resistance. There are people who cannot easily shift between the multiple realities of the transference, the therapeutic setting, and the (objective) characteristics of the therapist. These patients cannot make use of the psychoanalytic setting as a container of illusions. Because they lack the capacity for creative transformations, the analyst remains someone who is one-dimensional, literal, and concrete; he is only what is "objectively" perceived. Such patients have great difficulty in moving from an ordinary situation to an extraordinary one and back again; that is, they have great difficulty in accepting the paradox of the coexistence of separate realities. This inability to handle frames and paradoxes may be accompanied by a deficit in the use of language, such as that described by McDougall (1980). She identified a group of analytic patients she termed "anti-analysands," whose use of language lacked metaphoric imagery and reflected a paucity of symbolic transformations, so that their inner life appeared to be empty, shallow, and depleted. As McDougall observed, such patients cannot demonstrate the interpenetration of primary and secondary process thinking, the intermingling of imagery, fantasy, and conscious thought.

In "Analysis Terminable and Interminable" (1937) Freud attributed the limitations placed upon the process of cure to such factors as the strength of the instincts and certain alterations of the ego, whether congenital or acquired. A relative or absolute incapacity for illusioning, for symbolic transformations, or for the appreciation of paradox would also fall under the heading of an alteration of the ego.

We do not have any definitive answers as to what differentiates those individuals who are able to handle paradox from those who are not. The acceptance of paradox and the capacity for creative illusioning are probably all of a piece. Winnicott has said that, from the standpoint of the subject, the transitional object *symbolizes the interplay of separateness and union*. Creativity cannot exist without this particular illusion.

If we believe that creativity is, in some fashion, dependent upon the interplay of separateness and union, we are confronted with a further question: how is separateness accepted? What is it that enables a patient to accept the analyst's separate construction of reality and transform it into something of his own? Winnicott provided a tenta-

tive answer regarding the child's acceptance of the mother's separateness in his paper "The Use of an Object and Relating through
Identifications" (1971). There he made the startling suggestion that
the acceptance of the externality, of the separateness of the object, is
supported by the mother's acceptance of the baby's hatred. Extrapo-
lating from his experience with adult patients in psychoanalysis, Winnicott believed that in order to experience both the limitation of
personal omnipotence and the acceptance of the separateness of the
object, the child must also have experienced intense hatred (maximum destructiveness) toward the mother and know that they have
both survived (Winnicott 1971, p. 92).

We may consider the corresponding hypothesis: that a patient's
capacity to handle paradox, to apperceive the multiple levels of reality within the therapeutic setup, also requires the interplay of separateness and union. The interplay of merging and separateness is not
threatening to those whose sense of their own separateness is not
questioned, to those who are secure enough to allow themselves to
play with a merging union with others. Such people have no difficulty
in apperceiving multiple levels of reality.

For some patients the externality of the object and corresponding
separateness of the self are only achieved when they experience, in
Winnicott's language, "maximum destructiveness" and know that
they and the analyst have survived. For these patients, experiencing
the point of maximum destructiveness with the assurance of mutual
survival may be a necessary developmental step within the treatment
before they can fully handle the paradox of transference.

Resistance and the Transformation of Psychic Pain

The therapeutic process inevitably generates a certain quantum of
psychic pain. Transference gratification may paradoxically result in
psychic pain and a mourning for a love that can never materialize;
deep, unsatisfied yearnings are reawakened only to be once again
thwarted. In the course of treatment one is inevitably confronted with
the painful fact of one's own limitations and the limitations of others;
one is confronted with the loss of future expectations and the unful-
fillment of old ideals. This discrepancy between the wished-for and
the actual self is inevitably painful (Joffe and Sandler 1965).

The experience of psychic pain is at bottom the experience of loss
(Freud 1926). Freud distinguished psychic pain from anxiety in that

the former is a response to actual loss, while anxiety is a reaction to the danger that the loss would entail. Pontalis (1981) proposed that psychic pain occupied a *middle* position: halfway between anxiety and mourning. But unlike anxiety, which is communicable, psychic pain belongs only to oneself. One may cry out in pain, but the cry does not assuage. In this sense psychic pain is noncommunicable, but it can be transformed into something else that can be communicated. This capacity for the transformation of psychic pain is allied to the capacity for creativity. As Stephen Spender noted (1986), the greatness of the artist consists of his capacity to translate the harsh, unpoetic material of the world into poetry. This capacity for the transformation of psychic pain may be present in those who are not particularly gifted but who possess what might be called a creative attitude toward life. Might it be possible that psychic pain in the creative individual acts upon another level of reality and transforms it?

The experience of psychic pain can also serve as a major source of resistance. One may discern two completely opposite reactions to psychic pain, both of which are formidable obstacles to therapeutic change. In some patients there is an absolute avoidance of psychic pain, as if so much pain has already been experienced that desperate measures must be used to avoid a recurrence. In others there is an attachment to psychic pain, as if it were an addiction. Valenstein (1973) described patients who are attached to psychic pain to the extent that the pain itself contributes to a negative therapeutic reaction. In some patients there is an attachment to painful affect categories that represent a painful interaction with members of the nuclear family. It is as if the pain represents the person, so that to give up the pain may be experienced as an act of disloyalty; this type of attachment to psychic pain is a kind of perverse nostalgia. Thus the attachment to psychic pain impedes the recontextualization of time. As a form of trauma, it results in a foreshortening of present and future time in favor of time past.

8

The Patient's Use of
the Therapist

It has long been evident that every patient makes use of the therapeutic process in his own distinctive fashion. The therapist may have her own hopes and expectations regarding the use the patient will make of the treatment, but it is always the patient who decides.[1] The implication here is that there is also a wisdom of the mind that parallels the wisdom of the body, as in the observation that young children will, if left to their own devices, choose a diet that will ensure their survival. The use that the patient makes of the analyst will, in part, govern whether the knowledge acquired through the therapeutic experience will be transitory or lasting; whether learning from the therapeutic experience will be an "as-if" vicarious borrowing of the analyst's consciousness, or knowledge that becomes a permanent part of the self.

There is also a sense in which the acquisition of knowledge is analogous to forms of loving.[2] One may acquire knowledge through love of an earlier tradition, or knowledge may be completely self-created. There are also forms of knowing that appear to be self-created but are dependent upon the seed planted by others. A fertilizing idea may be borrowed from another person, as Freud borrowed from Breuer, but afterward when the seed is transformed the other person may become dispensable. In some cases the acquisition of knowledge may require the continued presence, support, and affirmation of the other person. As in modes of loving, the other person may be passive and unobtrusive or may be an active and equal partner.

This diversity of the use that is made of the therapeutic process might require equally diverse theories of therapeutic action, correlated to different stages of development or diagnostic groupings.[3] I propose another strategy: that the patient's use of the analyst is correlated with dynamically changing states of object-relatedness. For a correlation between the patient's use of the therapist and a character diagnosis is unsatisfactory because the use made of the therapist will alter as the treatment progresses.[4]

In the previous chapter I described the various forms of resistance that interfere with the process of recontextualizing unassimilated experiences, such as the inability to handle paradox, the addiction to or avoidance of psychic pain, and the schizoid defense of self-sufficiency that may preclude learning from others. Resistance can also be thought of as a description of the use that is made of the therapist.

This utilization of the therapist reflects *modes of relatedness* that have a certain developmental significance in that it is possible to refer to "higher" and "lower" levels of relatedness. I tend to think of object-relatedness as a characterological plateau from which there can be unexpected ascents and descents. But in thinking of modes of object-relatedness, I do not wish to imply anything that is uniform or orderly with points of closure, but rather something that is fluid and dynamic. The theory of *Nachträglichkeit* eliminates the idea that developmental stages have sharply defined beginnings and endings.[5]

Winnicott proposed in his paper "The Use of an Object and Relating through Identifications" (1969)[6] that the use of an object, which is linked to the object's externality, requires that the object be beyond the reach of the subject's omnipotent control. The recognition of the externality of the object requires, as noted earlier, an experience of "maximum destructiveness" with the assurance that both self and object have survived. In that paper Winnicott distinguishes *relating* to an object from the *use* of an object. This I believe creates a certain terminological confusion in that I consider *relating* to be a more inclusive, generic term. The use of an object must also be considered as a mode of relating. What Winnicott intended to convey is that relating to an object begins at birth, but use of an object occurs only after a certain developmental step has been taken. These stages of the use made of the object can be thought of as an organizational state of the ego. I intend to depict three such modes or levels of relatedness: (1) the dehumanization of the object (Winnicott's stage of preconcern); (2) self-containment in a state of contiguity (the sphere within the sphere); (3) shared creativity that results from an interplay of separateness and merging.

The Dehumanization of the Therapist

Winnicott characterized a developmental stage of *preconcern* in his paper "The Development of the Capacity for Concern" (1963). This paper can be thought of as an addendum to Melanie Klein's concept of the *paranoid-schizoid position,* which Winnicott rightly judged to be an unfortunate term. As portrayed by Klein, the paranoid-schizoid position is a stage in which the personhood of the object remains unperceived and unacknowledged, and accordingly the guilt that is evoked by the impulse to destroy the object is not experienced. The experience of guilt awaits the development of the *depressive position.* Segal (1981) makes the important point that the term *position* refers to a state of *organization* of the ego; such an organizational state would include the self as well as the object. In keeping with this line of thought, Winnicott proposed that there can be a dissociation in the child's ego so that the mother is split into an *object-mother* and an *environmental-mother.* These terms never became established, but what I believe Winnicott was attempting to portray is that the mother can function as a protective environment and at the same time be exploited as a non-person.

Similarly, the patient may believe that the therapist does not have any needs of his own, that the therapist is simply a functional entity performing a task without feelings, that the therapist is an inanimate tool at the patient's disposal. This dehumanization of the therapist is often rationalized by patients as consistent with what they believe to be the natural, expectable, and necessary *modus operandi* of the therapeutic process. The dehumanization of the therapist can be dissociated from other functions, in the manner suggested by Winnicott's dissociated object-mother and environmental-mother: at the same time the therapist is dehumanized, he can also be used as a protective environment, as a container of noxious affects, as a source of judicious observations, as a guide to unconscious motives, and so forth. Not surprisingly, this dehumanized mode of relatedness leads to the exploitation of the therapist. The dehumanization of the therapist reflects a unidimensional, one-level view of reality; the therapist is perceived *only* within the frame and not as a person in ordinary life, as illustrated in the following anecdote.

On one occasion an analytic hour was interrupted by a phone call informing me of a medical emergency involving my wife. I told my patient in a regretful manner that I had to leave because of a personal emergency. He responded as follows: "I suspect that something happened to your wife, and if that is true I hope that she dies!" I was shocked by the ferocity of his assault on me and the apparent lack of guilt and human concern. Later, when we were able to examine this episode, I learned that his fury at being interrupted was similar to the fury he expressed toward his mother, who permitted him to treat her as a "thing" to be used and to whom he reacted furiously when his needs were not met. This was a role in which she colluded: he thought of her as having no needs or desires of her own. Similarly, he did not think that I would be injured by his response because he believed that analysts were above such feelings. Much later, when he was no longer in this stage of preconcern, he experienced a delayed guilt reaction regarding his assault on me and wanted to make reparation. Winnicott suggested that the concern for the object, which includes the capacity to experience guilt, is facilitated if the baby has a contribution to make to the environment-mother; this relieves the anxiety that the mother will be consumed. The mother of this patient did not easily accept his love, and this situation was repeated with me when his reparative offering, a tip on the stock market, was a gift that I could not accept.

The stage of preconcern is also illustrated in this interchange with another patient. This episode occurred at the end of an extremely difficult analysis with a woman who was nearly mute. Although there were some therapeutic gains, the psychoanalysis could not be judged to be successful. In the last hours before termination, as we were assessing the treatment and its results, I acknowledged that it had been a very difficult treatment for both of us. She responded: "Why did *you* find it difficult? You were paid!" When I explored this statement further, I discovered that her disbelief that her treatment could also have been difficult for me was not expressed simply out of anger; she literally believed it to be true. She could not even conceive of the possibility that I had made any special effort on her behalf or that I had tried to do anything for her beyond what was included within a strict definition of my job. As in the other anecdote, I was dehumanized and considered only as a utilitarian object. In both cases, there was an absence of the apperception of multiple levels of reality. Instead, there was only the monolithic reality of the frame; there was no perception of me as an ordinary person with feelings, needs, and desires.

Being Alone in the Presence of the Therapist

In Chapter 7 I described another mode of relatedness as a sphere within a sphere. From one direction it can be viewed as a state of resistance, but from another direction it is a state that promotes healing. The patient remains within her self-contained cocoon, yet she is being held by the larger sphere of the therapeutic setting. The therapeutic setting can be thought of as an outer shell or a second skin that protects the analysand from the external world while still allowing the preservation of her construction of reality. As I described earlier, in the absence of an adequate parental holding environment the child's self-created world is necessary for survival; it is a measure born out of intense need, out of a state of emergency where psychic survival is at stake. For a child to rely only on itself for its safety in the world it must depend upon fantasies of omniscience and omnipotent control. When such fantasies are at the center of the self, they may be judged to be the consequence of an environmental emergency. The safety of the therapeutic environment may, of course, offer a second chance, a chance to create an inner world that is not a response to an environmental danger. It is a chance to discover one's personal life, to have one's own thoughts in a protected environment. But as Winnicott observed, it is paradoxical that the child learns to be alone in the presence of another. For some patients the use of the couch and the absence of visual contact with the analyst promote the illusion of being alone while still being aware of the analyst's presence.

In the psychoanalysis of the so-called narcissistic personality this mode of relatedness may exist for years. The essential point for these patients is that *the analysand's private world may or may not be shared with the analyst, but the analyst's construction of reality should not intrude upon this private world.* It is for this reason that Balint, Winnicott, and Kohut have all warned, each in his own characteristic fashion, of the dangers of the analyst's intrusion. Balint (1968) said:

> The last train of thought is connected with my ideas about the area of creation, an area of the mind in which there is no external orga-

nized object, and any intrusion of such an object by attention-seeking interpretations inevitably destroys for the patient the possibility of creating something out of himself (p. 176) . . . the analyst—must not be felt as in any way demanding, interfering, intruding, as this would reinforce the old oppressive inequality between subject and object (p. 180).

Winnicott offered similar advice (1971, p. 57): "My description amounts to a plea to every therapist to allow for the patient's capacity to play, that is, to be creative in the analytic work. The patient's creativity can be only too easily stolen by a therapist who knows too much."

When patients are in a mode of self-holding, empathy is the least intrusive form of intervention inasmuch as it is essentially a mirror of the patient's constructed reality. Winnicott has advised that it is important to wait before making interpretations—to let the patient "simply be." Kohut, who places the use of empathy at the center of his theory of treatment (the theory of the selfobject), recognizes the same therapeutic principle of the need for non-intrusion and of the healing effect of empathy that mirrors the contents of the analysand's inner world. Kohut's selfobject is, as the term signifies, an object that mirrors the self, an object that does not introduce another constructed reality. Kohut claims (1984, p. 66) that "the gradual acquisition of empathic contact with mature selfobjects is the essence of the psychoanalytic cure." He further states that the step that defines the psychoanalytic cure is "the opening of a path of empathy between self and selfobjects, specifically the establishment of empathic intuneness between self and selfobjects on mature adult levels. This new channel of empathy permanently takes the place of the formerly repressed or split-off archaic narcissistic relationship: it supplants the bondage that had formerly tied the archaic self to the archaic selfobject."

Kohut's clearest definition of the term *selfobject* occurs in a letter to a colleague (1984, p. 52):

Throughout his life a person will experience himself as a cohesive harmonious firm unit in time and space, connected with his past and pointing meaningfully into a creative-productive future, [but] only as long as, at each stage in his life, he experiences certain representatives of his human surroundings as joyfully responding to him, as available to him as sources of idealized strength and calmness, as being silently present but in essence like him, and, at any rate, able to grasp his inner life more or less accurately so that their responses are attuned to his needs and allow him to grasp their inner life when he is in need of such sustenance.

Kohut's description of the use of a selfobject reminds me of the artist's use of a muse.[7] The muse is there only for the subject and does not intrude with her own needs and desires; a muse supports the creativity of the subject by affirming and consolidating, through empathy, the subject's construction of reality, a reality that is not to be challenged. Kohut's selfobject, however, unlike Winnicott's environment-mother or the sphere within the sphere, is not a second skin or an alternative protective environment.

Shared Creativity: The Interplay of Separateness and Merging Union

If the patient makes use of the analyst only as a selfobject, reflecting back what is already known, there may be a strengthening of the sense of self, but the patient will not profit from the knowledge of the *analyst's* construction of reality. The analyst must also be free to introduce, by means of interpretation, that which is novel and unexpected. If the patient's sense of self is not threatened, he will welcome the analyst's creativity and not experience it as an intrusion. This mode of relatedness, which may be present in the "healthier" patient at the start of treatment, represents a higher level of development for those who do not have this capacity. This state of relatedness requires *the ability to merge playfully with the analyst yet retain a sense of separateness*. This is quite different from an archaic wish/fear of merger that is associated with giving up autonomy and being controlled, submerged, or swallowed up by the object. One can distinguish archaic from mature states of merging in that in the latter, the sense of separateness is maintained so that merging coexists with individuation. Playful merging will be impeded if there is a split-off, dissociated part of the self that retains fantasies of omnipotent control of the object.

It has long been recognized that psychotherapy is akin to a creative process. For Otto Rank (1978), the goal of both psychotherapy and the creative act was individuation. Rothenberg (1988) considers the sudden appearance or flash of insight as the result of a creative process, a synthesis of opposites that he called "Janusian." For Winnicott, playing and creativity are nearly interchangeable ideas; the aim of therapy is bringing a patient who is not able to play into a state of being able to play (1971, p. 31). For Winnicott the essence of creative perception rests on this interplay between separateness and merging. This can be illustrated by recalling Winnicott's squiggle game, which is fundamentally a game of shared creativity. It is a game in which Winnicott first makes a squiggle drawing and then the child turns it into something; then the child makes a squiggle and Winnicott turns it into something. By analogy, the patient presents a dream, which, although it is the patient's product, is also an object for both patient and analyst. The patient associates to the dream; the analyst focuses upon and interprets a particular element of the dream because of its affective charge; the patient then produces fresh associations, which in turn evokes further interpretation; and so on. In the end one may not know who made the interpretation. In Winnicott's potential space, one does not ask: whose reality is it? In this mode of relatedness there is no need to defend against intrusion.[8]

Winnicott believed that creativity begins at birth (1988, p. 101): [that] "the mother makes it possible for the baby to have the illusion that the breast has been created by impulse out of need." The mother's sensitivity will reinforce the baby's illusion of magical control of the breast. This experience of primary creativity provides a core that remains the foundation for a continuing positive attitude toward external reality. But a creative potential cannot rest simply upon this gratifying experience with the mother, for there is nothing to suggest that such gratifying experiences characterize the early life of creative individuals. What I find of greater relevance for the understanding of creativity is Winnicott's theory of the potential space. As noted earlier, Winnicott's potential space is a paradigm for the shared creativity that occurs when there is the capacity for playful merging and separateness. In this shared creativity, we do not ask: "Whose reality is it?" Winnicott has said that from the standpoint of the subject, *the transitional object symbolizes the interplay of separateness and union.* I believe this to be the essence of creativity; creativity cannot exist without this particular illusion.

When Winnicott (1969) addressed the question of how the child moves from a more archaic sense of merging to a state of playful merging, he suggested that the acceptance of the externality and of the separateness of the object is supported by the mother's acceptance of the baby's hatred. Let us consider the corresponding hypothesis: that a patient's capacity to handle paradox, to apperceive the multiple levels of reality within the therapeutic setup, also requires this capac-

ity for separateness and union. The interplay of merging and separateness is not threatening to those who have a firm sense of the self,
who are secure enough to allow themselves to play with a merging
union with others. Such people have no difficulty in apperceiving
multiple levels of reality.

The means by which a patient is "raised" to a higher level of
relatedness rest upon at least two separate but perhaps related processes. One includes all that contributes to individuation and the
strengthening of the patient's sense of self; the other refers to the
"borrowing" of the analyst's consciousness. The latter process is
more familiarly known under the heading of the *therapeutic alliance,*
which I shall discuss in the following section.

It has been my thesis that patients, if given the opportunity, will
select and recreate in the interaction with their therapist those elements that they require to complete the process of growth and individuation. That is to say, each patient will make use of the therapeutic
process in his own particular fashion. For this reason we must recognize that there are great variations in the path that patients travel in
order to strengthen their sense of self. All of our therapeutic en-
deavors aim at strengthening the sense of self and fostering individuation, but there are more specific therapeutic interactions that enable a
patient to experience a playful merging with the therapist without a
loss of individuation. Some patients require a gradual disillusionment
of fantasies of omnipotence of the self and of the object. Such omnipotent fantasies of the self arise, as I have said, as emergency measures when the child perceives the absence of a parental holding
environment. These fantasies may be split-off and dissociated, which
contributes to a loss of a sense of the wholeness and integrity of the
self. Such individuals vacillate between the experience of an inflated
grandiose self and a depleted helpless self, where the grandiosity is
attributed to the object. For these patients, the analyst's failure to
understand may be disillusioning, as a child is disillusioned when he
discovers that the parent cannot detect a lie (Kohut 1984). But to
recognize the limitations of the analyst's omniscience leads ultimately
to a strengthening of the self. Kohut describes this as structure build-
ing, as *optimal frustration;* Gedo (1988) speaks of the benefits of
optimal disillusionment.

Other patients may cling to an archaic illusion of merger with an
omniscient analyst who does not need to be told anything because he

already knows, as a mother anticipates the infant's or young child's needs without the child having to communicate. I have the impression that many patients need to provide themselves with a necessary experience of disillusionment with the analyst. For this reason, they may need to create an analyst who does not understand by unconsciously providing confusing or misleading information or by not providing the necessary clues.

In some cases patients sense that they are ready to move to a higher level of object-relatedness. The situation is analogous to that of a child who needs the parent to be able to respond to her changing level of development. I believe that in some instances the analyst's growing impatience with the analysand is ready to move to such a higher level of relatedness. Other patients need to recreate Winnicott's point of maximum destructiveness; that is, they need to recreate the experience of the externality of the analyst who is beyond omnipotent control. But in order for the patient's anger to promote growth, she must be beyond the stage of preconcern, which means that she must possess the capacity to experience guilt toward the analyst. This is why rage in borderline patients will not necessarily enable them to achieve a higher level of object-relatedness.

Comments on the Therapeutic Alliance

The patient's use of the therapist calls to mind the more familiar concept of the therapeutic alliance. Often a term that initially describes a technical process becomes separated from its original psychoanalytic context and is loosely applied as a descriptive term to a broad range of very different therapeutic encounters, such as the psychotherapy of the borderline states.[9] Such has been the fate of the term *therapeutic alliance*. It was initially intended to denote the state of collaboration that exists between analyst and analysand: whether the two participants share the aims, goals, and actual work of the treatment. The term *therapeutic alliance* is associated with Zetzel's *contribution* (1958, 1970) and is nearly synonymous with Greenson's term (1967) *working alliance*.[10] Despite the widespread use of the term, the underlying concept of the therapeutic alliance remains controversial. I believe that the source of this controversy can be traced to opposing theories of the therapeutic action of psychoanalysis: theories that can be described as classical or structural on one hand, and theories of treatment derived from an object-relations model on the other. (These different theories of therapeutic action will be discussed further in Chapter 10.)

Freud recognized that an alliance existed between the analyst and the patient against the common enemy, the patient's neurosis. This alliance can also be thought of as part of the unobjectionable positive transference which Freud differentiated from the transference neurosis. In "An Outline of Psychoanalysis" Freud speaks of a pact or an alliance that the analyst makes with the patient against the enemy (the instinctual demands of the id and the conscientious demands of the superego). Freud likened the situation to a civil war that requires the assistance of an outside ally (1940, p. 173):

> The analytic physician and the patient's weakened ego, basing themselves on the real external world, have to band themselves together into a party against the enemies, . . . the instinctual demands of the id and the conscientious demands of the super-ego. The sick ego promises us the most complete candor—promises, that is, to put at our disposal all the material which its self-perception yields it; we assure the patient of the strictest discretion and place at his service our experience in interpreting material that has been influenced by the unconscious. Our knowledge is to make up for his ignorance and to give his ego back its mastery over lost provinces of his mental life. This pact constitutes the analytic situation.

The concept of the therapeutic alliance owes a great deal to Sterba's paper "The Fate of the Ego in the Analytic Therapy" (1934). Sterba's contribution is an elaboration of Freud's position to which he adds the novel idea of a therapeutic dissociation or split within the patient's ego that corresponds to an analogous dissociation within the analyst's ego. Sterba describes in effect the analysand's "borrowing" the analyst's consciousness, especially with reference to the split between the observing and the experiencing ego. As in Vygotsky's zone of proximal development, the analyst serves the learner as a vicarious form of consciousness until such time as the patient is able to master his own consciousness. Sterba also describes the analyst's detachment in the face of the analysand's passion, which enables the analysand to gain mastery over his instinctual life. Sterba notes that an interpretation leads to a "new point of view of intellectual contemplation" which is disjunctive with immediate experience. Although the analyst's consciousness, that is to say, the analytic attitude, has its own special attributes, it is, in a broader sense, a descendant of the ancient principle of introspection. William James's description of introspection as a *stream of consciousness* (1890) observed a similar dissociation in that the continuous stream of consciousness is interrupted by the observing mind observing itself.

Sterba's description remains essentially intrapsychic. The importance of Zetzel's concept of the therapeutic alliance is that Sterba's observing and experiencing ego is brought into the two-person context of the object relationship that exists between therapist and patient. Zetzel's contribution was threefold: first, she reaffirmed Freud's distinction between the transference neurosis and the unobjectionable positive transference; second, in separating the therapeutic alliance from the transference neurosis she underlined the importance of what is now called the psychoanalytic setting, tracing its origins to an early mother-child relationship; and finally, she emphasized that the therapeutic alliance is an *object relationship* (in current time, in the here and now) based in part on the "real" or "human" qualities of the analyst.

Zetzel's therapeutic alliance, like Sterba's therapeutic dissociation, depends upon the analysand's "borrowing" from the analyst a fundamental attitude concerning their work together. This attitude goes beyond the analyst's introspection in that it is communicated by demonstration. It is in this way that an early interpretation of the transference demonstrates the analyst's appreciation of the existence of multiple levels of reality. Thus, *the analyst's demonstration of the paradoxical coexistence of multiple levels of reality is implicit in the therapeutic alliance.* Zetzel (1958) illustrated her concept by means of the following case material taken from supervision. An inexperienced and anxious candidate with his first analytic patient behaved in a rigid, aloof, and silent manner, lest any activity be regarded as unanalytic. This greatly contributed to the anxiety of his patient, who thought of him as a distant, Olympian, magical figure. The supervisor in effect gave the analyst permission to behave in a more human manner, and as a result the analysand realized that the picture of him had been fantastic, that he was after all "an ordinary man" (p. 190). I believe this vignette illustrates that the student analyst had not understood the paradox that to function as an analyst within the frame does not preclude one's presence as an ordinary person. The more experienced analyst is able to shift effortlessly from one level of reality to another so that this paradox is taken for granted. *The analytic attitude includes the acceptance of the paradox of the coexistence of the asymmetric relation within the frame and the egalitarian relationship outside of the frame.*

Zetzel's concept of the therapeutic alliance has been criticized by some analysts, such as Brenner (1979) and Friedman (1969). Brenner sees Zetzel's recommendation that the analyst should behave in a more "human" fashion to be a manipulation that introduces an undesirable form of gratification, as if the therapeutic alliance were an example of a "corrective emotional experience" in contrast to "correct understanding and consistent interpretation" (1979, p. 146). Brenner also disagrees with Zetzel's assertion that the therapeutic alliance is not a form of transference; Brenner does not see any distinction between the therapeutic alliance and the transference neurosis.[11] Friedman (1969), in a broadly based review of the concept of the therapeutic alliance, also criticized it as an unwarranted form of maternal gratification but pointedly omitted any reference to Zetzel's contribution. I believe that this criticism of the concept of the therapeutic alliance reflects a more fundamental disagreement concerning the premises of the theories of object relations, a topic that will be explored in Chapter 10.

9

Paradox and Therapeutic Dilemmas

The pervasiveness of paradox within the psychoanalytic process has been a leitmotif of this work. It should be noted, however, that I have been using the term *paradox* only in a descriptive sense, defining it as a contradictory phenomenon that is fundamentally true. I must leave it to others to judge whether the psychology of paradox bears any relation to the analysis of paradox to be found in formal and mathematical logic.[1]

As I noted in the previous chapter, William James (1890) observed an important paradox: the continuity that characterizes the stream of consciousness is interrupted by observation; there is a disjunction between the experiencing and the observing mind. Gerald Holton (1973), a historian of science, traced how James's observation of this disjunction, the complementarity of the mind observing its own experience, provided the seed that led Niels Bohr to apply the idea of complementarity to quantum mechanics. Bohr acknowledged his indebtedness to psychology and to William James in particular (Holton 1973). In noting the analogy between atomic physics and human psychology, he suggested that paradox may be central to human psychology as it is to atomic physics (Bohr 1958, p. 27): "In introspection, it is clearly impossible to distinguish sharply between the phenomena themselves and their conscious perception . . . it will appear on closer examination that we really have to do in such cases with *mutually exclusive* situations" (my emphasis).

Freud has often been criticized for the inconsistencies that can be uncovered in his texts. Accordingly, he has been identified by various authors as a biologist of the mind; as a moralist; as a humanist; and so forth. This multifaceted complexity reflects, I believe, not only Freud's character but also the paradoxical nature of the human mind. I am not among those who believe that Freud was always right, but I do think that he intuitively grasped that paradox is intrinsic to the human mind and that to force observations into a unitary system will destroy the essence of understanding. Hannah Arendt (quoted in Draenos 1982, p. 8) made an important observation that pertains to Freud's inconsistencies: "Fundamental and flagrant contradictions rarely occur in second-rate writers, in whom they can be discounted, in the work of great authors they lead into the very center of their work and are the most important clue to a true understanding of their problems and new insights."

I believe then that Freud sensed the paradox implicit in mental phenomena but chose not to make it explicit. I suspect that he believed that to emphasize paradox would be incompatible with his (nineteenth-century) view of science. Had Freud known that paradox was at the heart of quantum mechanics, he might not have hesitated to identify explicitly the paradox of transference. As mentioned earlier, he saw transference love as something that was real and at the same time unreal; the transference neurosis was understood to be a repetition of the past and at the same time a newly created illness; transference is the major resistance to recovery and at the same time the motor that generates the cure. We can add further to this list: because of the idiosyncratic qualities of the two participants, transference is a happening, yet the fact that transference is a repeatable configuration, derived from psychic structure, makes it possible to utilize the transference as a nosological marker. The paradox of time, that the past can alter the present and the present can alter the past, is also implicit in Freud's idea of *Nachträglichkeit*. Freud never integrated this deep awareness of the paradox of time into his theory of transference.

In his introduction to "Playing and Reality" Winnicott made a plea that paradox be accepted, tolerated, and respected (1971, p. xii). The theory of the transitional object also rests on a paradox: that we do not ask the infant or child whether the transitional object was created by the child or presented from without. Winnicott's paradox of the transitional object rests on the presence and interpenetration of multiple levels of reality: an external object is transformed by means of the child's inner reality. This illusionary space, Winnicott's potential space in which playing takes place, is also real and not-real. My description of a particular mode of object-relatedness, the sphere within the sphere, is derived from a different Winnicottian paradox, that the capacity to be alone requires the presence of the mother.

Gregory Bateson introduced the theory of the double bind into psychiatry. It is a theory of paradoxical communication in which the formal, paradoxical aspects of certain communications, not their content, make an appropriate response impossible. This was proposed initially as a contribution to the etiology of schizophrenia. Anzieu (1986), following Bateson, observed similar paradoxical communications leading to double binds in transference and countertransference phenomena in psychoanalysis, which he termed *paradoxical transference*. An example of a paradoxical communication that is relevant for certain therapeutic dilemmas in psychoanalysis, which I shall consider shortly, is the request implicit in the fundamental rule: *Be spontaneous!*[2] Bateson also made the important prediction that, in the case of certain individuals, their psychopathology will consist of an inability to accept paradox, to accept the paradox of the concurrent existence of that which is within the frame and that which is outside. I have described the inability to handle paradox as a form of resistance. The capacity to apperceive paradox, is, I believe, a function of a "higher" mode of object-relatedness in which there is an effortless transition between separateness and merging union. Ivrim Kumin (1978) also sees the acceptance of paradox as a higher developmental function. There is, he believes, a pervasive fear of paradox, and he suggests that the defensive splitting of the ego may be the child's means of reconciling intolerable paradox.

Recognizing that the presence of multiple levels of reality creates paradox clarifies certain observations regarding transference that might otherwise seem confusing. The recognition of paradox leads to the acceptance of the idea that the psychoanalytic setting, something that is "real" in the sense that it is here in present time, can also symbolically actualize aspects of the earliest stages of a mother-child relationship. Recognizing the fundamentally paradoxical nature of transference allows us to clarify the concept of regression in the transference and sheds new light on the controversy over whether transference is a repetition of the past or whether it is something in the here and now. This controversy reflects divergent theoretical convictions: there are those who interpret transference repetition as evidence of the validity of Freud's instinct theory, and others who reject instinct theory in favor of an interpersonal theory that supports the view that transference is in the here and now. Transference as repetition and transference in the here and now can now be seen as *complementary* levels of reality analogous to the complementarity of the wave and the particle.

In *Psychoanalysis in a New Context* (Modell 1984a) I described the paradox of the self concept that is revealed in Freud's terminological vacillation between *ego* and *self*. The self concept belongs to both a one-person and a two-person psychology; the self is defined as a developmental structure that can only be modified slowly, but the experience of self can be evanescent and can change rapidly in response to another person or to the image of the self that is reflected by the response of a group. The paradox of the self is not only that the self is both permanent and transient but that it is something that is also both hidden and social. The self is a social entity; Harry Stack Sullivan (1950) once stated that inasmuch as the self is defined by others, individuals do not exist. Yet the self is partly hidden from others, and parts of the self may also be hidden and split off from one's own conscious awareness. Lichtenstein (1963, p. 199) observed this same paradox in Erikson's identity concept: "Any definable identity requires that we perceive ourselves as objects, which means equating identity with the identity given to us as social roles, losing thereby the sense of identity as pure actuality of being."

Wherever we look at the self concept we meet paradox. We should expect, therefore, that this paradox will engender dilemmas for both therapist and patient. Anzieu (1986) commented that the logic of paradox is at the foundation of the deficit in narcissistic and borderline patients. The dilemmas that are associated with disorders of the self reflect a different logic from that of intrapsychic conflict. In contemplating this problem we encounter terminological difficulties, for we do not have a recognized term that differentiates resolvable conflict from the conflicts embedded in dilemmas to which there may be no resolution.[3]

Most therapeutic dilemmas are never really resolved; they merely become less significant when the patient achieves a higher level of object-relatedness. Kohut (1977), for very different reasons, has claimed that self psychology is not a psychology of conflict. But as I and others have noted, this view cannot be sustained.[4] For the dilemmas associated with disturbances of the self can become intensely conflictual. One has only to think of the central dilemma of schizoid people: that closeness to others threatens the existence and continuity of the self, yet withdrawal leads to a sense of deadness that ultimately may threaten the individual's attachment to reality. I believe that Kohut's theory has led to a mistaken polarity between deficiency states and states of conflict, but there are subtle differences between disturbances of the sense of self and intrapsychic conflict that follow from the paradoxical nature of the self.

The Dilemma of Non-Communication

If the sphere within the sphere is a mode of object-relatedness in which the therapist is used as a selfobject muse that strengthens and reinforces the patient's faith in his creative apperception, any activity on the therapist's part that is not in keeping with this muse-like function may be experienced as an unwelcome intrusion that interrupts the continuity of the sense of self. Thus, the analyst's construction of the patient's inner reality, unless it is nearly synchronous with that inner reality, may be felt as an intrusion, or, as Glover (1955) noted, as a suggestion. Such suggestions may carry an implicit message that the analysand should submit to the analyst's superior knowledge.

Inasmuch as we can only understand our patients through what is communicated to us, when the patient is essentially talking to himself in our presence, we may become restless and wish to get on with the treatment and thus deal with this as a resistance. Recall that this mode of object-relatedness is intrinsically paradoxical in that viewed from one direction it is a resistance, but when seen from a different perspective it is a curative form of self-holding in the protective presence of the analyst. If the therapist chooses to treat this as a resistance, he may interfere with the healing of the self; if he simply lets the patient be, that is, accepts the self-holding, he may not enable the patient to achieve a higher mode of relatedness. Responding to the non-communication as resistance may be experienced by the patient as an invasion of the privacy of the self; ignoring the resistance may impede the progress of the treatment. Such dilemmas present the therapist with a no-win situation.

The therapist's problem is to decide when to act and when to let the patient simply be. The therapist always needs to discern whether the patient wishes to be known or wishes to maintain his privacy. There are times when the patient may be desperately in need of being rescued from his isolation. This state of affairs may shift within a given hour or may extend for a matter of months if not years. Such situations require all of the therapist's experience and intuition to determine the patient's genuine needs as opposed to his defensive enactments. Therapeutic dilemmas that arise from the paradoxical logic of the self will not simply yield to interpretation, but the therapist's insight in recognizing and accepting the dilemma is essential.

The Therapist's Agenda

The therapist's desire to overcome the patient's non-communication so that he or she can better understand the patient and thus further the goals of the treatment is part of the larger issue of the therapist's agenda. The therapeutic dilemma here is perhaps as old as psychotherapy itself. It is the dilemma that is implicit in the use of authority and power, such as the hypnotist's power of suggestion. We know that the role of the therapist as well as the goals of the treatment cannot be completely separated from cultural values. In the nineteenth century, physicians could easily assume the role of an authoritative father, but today the arbitrary use of authority by the physician is unacceptable. The patient-physician relationship, at least in this country, has become more egalitarian; the patient is now viewed by society as a consumer with a right to know and a right to be informed.

The aims of treatment are also influenced by cultural values, such as the quest for autonomy and self-actualization,[5] which are imported into the goals of psychotherapy and psychoanalysis. In our antiauthoritarian contemporary social context the therapist says in effect: "In order to achieve a greater measure of self-actualization, you must *submit* yourself to my superior knowledge and experience." It is a variant of the command: *Be spontaneous!* Of course the therapist must possess superior knowledge, but the superiority is limited to the therapist's function within the frame. For those patients who can handle paradox this presents no problem; but others have difficulty in accepting the paradox of the coexistence of these two different levels of reality—the absence of equality within the frame and the equality that exists outside of the frame.[6] Where there is a significant impairment of the integrity of the self, leading to the defense we call schizoid—and many of us are schizoid to some degree—submission to the therapist's agenda is experienced as a demand for compliance, a repetition of an earlier submissive compliance to parental agendas.

This becomes a particular problem for those individuals who believe that they were not loved for themselves and therefore that being loved was conditional upon their compliance. Conforming to the therapist's agenda confirms their conviction that an object relationship, by definition, means being controlled, subjugated, and ultimately swallowed up by the other person. For such patients, that one can be in a relationship with another human being and still retain one's autonomy is simply unbelievable.

For all these reasons, it is essential that we not impose our agenda on our patients. We all know that we try not to impose our moral values on our patients, but nevertheless we retain certain convictions regarding the aims of treatment that exist as an explicit or implicit agenda. But is it not foolish to assert that the therapist should be *without* a plan, without certain goals and expectations that she wishes to achieve? One is reminded here of Bion's aphorism that the therapist should be without memory or desire. This prescription is like an impossible Zen koan; but it does contain a measure of truth. What Bion is recommending is that the analyst be non-attached:[7] for the analyst to be too attached to the goals of treatment will be counterproductive. By desiring more one obtains less; the therapist's agenda is more likely to be realized in a state of non-attachment. King made the same observation when she said (1962, p. 227): "I would therefore suggest that this attitude of 'non-attachment' (to use a term from Eastern philosophy) is a crucial factor in the curative process, and one of our main therapeutic tools in our attempt to help our patients to live in their own present, unmolested by unresolved infantile conflicts."

Yet can the therapist be non-attached? We also know of the importance of the analyst's vision of her patient in the *future*. As Loewald (1980) described in his paper "On the Therapeutic Action of Psychoanalysis," a mature parental object relation consists of an ability to relate to the child in accordance with his shifting levels of development. Although there is a time when it is necessary for the analyst to let the patient be, it is also necessary that the analyst have some sense of what the patient can *become*. That is to say, it is important that we not accept our patients at their lowest level of functioning.

We desire to be useful to our patients and if possible to relieve them of suffering. Although "maturity" may constitute a cultural value, it is difficult to avoid the conclusion that in some instances the patient's suffering is the result of a failure to accept the limitations of reality.

For ultimately, as Freud said, our alliance with the patient is based on "the real external world" (Freud 1940, p. 173). For some patients the analyst becomes, whether intentionally or not, a representative of the reality principle.

Thus the analyst is and is not without memory and desire. We cannot avoid the hope that our patient will achieve a higher level of object-relatedness within the treatment that will ultimately be relocated to a life outside of the treatment. As part of our "impossible profession" we must cope with the paradox of attachment and non-attachment to our therapeutic aims.

Ultimately, however, both therapist and patient will face certain requirements of the therapeutic process which will have to be met in some form or another. For the treatment to be effective, the patient must ultimately be able to communicate spontaneously and authentically. It is at this point that the therapist's agenda becomes explicit, and the patient is then free to either accept or reject it. This intervention has multiple meanings: it is an indication of the separateness that exists between the two participants, the separateness that coexists with merging contiguity; but perhaps more important, it is a symbolic reenactment of the fact that a relationship consists of two separate people, each with his or her separate desires and different views of reality. For the therapist to acknowledge his agenda, after an initial period of letting the patient be, indicates that a relationship is possible where both partners retain their autonomy and personhood, and that to share the therapist's agenda does not mean that the therapist will control the patient. That two people can be in a relationship in which the personhood and autonomy of the other are preserved and mutually respected will be, for some, a totally novel experience.

The Paradox of Transference Gratification

Freud's "principle" of abstinence—the extent to which gratification is experienced through the transference—also leads to therapeutic dilemmas. This point can be illustrated by recalling the transference paradigm in Chapter 3. There I described an analysand who said: "I want you to love me!" This sentence revealed the multiple levels of reality present in the psychoanalytic setting. The *I* who wants me to love her may refer to the patient in actuality, that is, as she is today, an adult woman. The *I* may, in addition, refer to another level of reality—not the Ms. X as she is in ordinary life but the Ms. X who is my patient; that is, Ms. X within the frame of the psychoanalytic setting. Or the *I* may be a reference to the little girl in Ms. X. Similarly, I described how the *you* referring to myself also contains at least three levels of reality: myself as an ordinary person; myself as an analyst (within the frame); and finally, the *you* might refer to an iconic representation of her father. Thus the words *I, you,* and *me* in the sentence "I want you to love me!" could, depending on their context, denote three different levels of reality: that of ordinary life; that of the analytic frame; and that of the iconic/projective transference. Given the presence of these multiple levels of reality, we can readily understand that abstinence and gratification will become paradoxical, since *gratification at any one level of reality leads to paradoxical frustration at another*. If the patient did experience love from me as a "real" object, this would disrupt the frame of the analysis; she would in effect lose the analysis. If I interpreted that her wish to be loved by me was *only* a displacement of her wish to be loved by her father, she might feel that such an observation was demeaning and rejecting, as if I were saying that this is *only* a transference reaction. If she experienced love from me as a father, the gratification would lead to an acute sense of loss because she would experience that her relation with her father is irretrievably gone.

Transference gratification has always been implicitly acknowledged to be paradoxical. Analysts have long recognized that, to the extent that the analytic relationship takes on the character of a relationship in ordinary life, this will preclude or inhibit the development of the transference. Strachey noted this when he said (1934, p. 285): "The patient's sense of reality has the narrowest limits. It is a paradoxical fact that the best way of ensuring that his ego shall be able to distinguish between phantasy and reality is to withhold reality from him as much as possible." For this reason we restrict our social contacts with our analysands, as we restrict the sharing of the kind of personal information that would be commonplace in a friendship. Yet if this process goes too far, if the analyst behaves *only* as an analyst and not as an ordinary human being, this will impede the development of a therapeutic alliance (Zetzel 1970). The analyst must demonstrate his capacity to shift easily from one level of reality to another, inasmuch as the analysand borrows or vicariously assumes the analyst's consciousness.[8] One wishes to facilitate a *contrast between different levels of reality*. This contrast between different levels of reality also requires a certain balance between abstinence and gratification. Fox

(1984) recognized the therapeutic dilemma of abstinence when he spoke of the need to "titrate" the analytic situation to maintain an optimal tension between gratification and withdrawal.

The "principle" of abstinence, as Freud indicated, does not refer only to sexual gratification (1915, pp. 164–165):

> I have already let it be understood that analytic technique requires of the physician that he should deny to the patient who is craving for love the satisfaction she demands. The treatment must be carried out in *abstinence* [my emphasis]. By this I do not mean physical abstinence alone, nor yet the deprivation of everything that the patient desires, for perhaps no sick person could tolerate this. Instead, I shall state it as a fundamental principle that the patient's needs and longings should be allowed to persist in her, in order that they may serve as forces impelling her to do work and to make changes,[9] and we must be aware of appeasing those forces by means of surrogates.

Yet Freud also said that the analysand's resistance is overcome only by means of love for the analyst. In this same paper Freud (1915) described the analysand's love for the analyst as only a proxy, which the analyst should not spoil by throwing a sausage on the track before the patient has finished the race.

The gratification that the patient experiences within the analytic relationship has been attributed to his dependency upon the analyst. Winnicott spoke of this as a "regression" to dependency. But there are, as Fairbairn reminded us, mature forms of dependency as well as infantile forms. Thus the term *dependency* appears to be too general and all-encompassing. For some individuals, dependency upon the analyst includes the creation of a beloved, subjectively created analyst who is a fantasy object and therefore can be omnipotently controlled. Living within the transference in this self-created reality may afford more satisfaction than living in the real world. This may be, to be sure, a "new" object relationship, but it may be like Freud's sausage on the track that prevents the patient from finishing the race.

Achieving Safety through the Experience of Danger

The therapeutic action of psychoanalysis and psychoanalytic psychotherapy results from the contrast between different levels of reality, inasmuch as the contrast between present objects and archaic objects furthers the retranscription of affect categories. This creates the paradox that the analyst represents the dangers of the past as well as the safety of the present. Before the analyst can be perceived as safe, he must first be experienced as dangerous. The theory of therapy proposed by Weiss and Sampson (1986) proposes that patients need to test the safety of the therapeutic setting by recreating, consciously and unconsciously, situations of danger. They believe that patients wish to disconfirm their pathogenic beliefs. Weiss and Sampson assume that patients come to treatment with the conscious and unconscious desire to master early conflicts, traumas, and anxieties by means of an attempt to establish *conditions of safety* (Eagle 1984). I agree with this formulation. The analyst must pass the patient's test, but the patient can only disconfirm his worst fear by means of experience. As Freud said (1912, p. 108), the patient's illness must be recreated "not as an event in the past but as a present-day force" and that "when all is said and done, it is impossible to destroy anyone *in absentia or in effigy.*"

In his discussion of Weiss and Sampson's contribution, Eagle notes that, in contrast to classical theory, they stress the therapeutic value of *action*. Thus action is not an inferior form of remembering, as Freud had believed, but goes to the heart of the therapeutic process. Eagle introduces the term *enactment*,[10] which is similar to what I have called *symbolic actualization*.

I believe that the analysand will determine by her own actions whether or not the analyst corresponds to her disavowed objects or to the disavowed parts of herself. For example, if an individual had parents who were nearly incapable of placing the needs of their child before their own needs, such a person, when in analysis, will be intent upon discovering whether or not this is true of the analyst. I recall an instance where, in the initial interview, a prospective analysand peremptorily demanded that I refrain from smoking during *her* analysis. At that time I smoked small cigars, and although I did not know the meaning of this woman's demand, I assented to her request. Later, during the course of the analysis, I learned that it was absolutely necessary that this patient discover whether I could forgo my own pleasures in favor of her needs. For she experienced both her parents as self-indulgent, selfish people who were incapable of giving up anything for the sake of their children. The conflict that this patient recreated, that between her needs and those of her caretakers, is a characteristic form of parent-offspring conflict that has been observed in many animal species, including primates. Robert Trivers, an evolutionary biologist, believes that when the offspring perceives its parent's self-interest, "the offspring cannot rely on its parents for disinterested guidance" (1985, p. 159).

As I noted in the previous chapter, self-serving needs enter into the construction of reality; thus, before the analysand can entrust herself to the analyst and accept his construction of reality, she may need to test the analyst by recreating a conflict of divergent needs.

10

Theories of Psychoanalytic Treatment

There are many competing theories of psychoanalytic treatment that can be grouped under a variety of headings. Three significant categories are as follows: (1) Freud's theory of psychoanalytic treatment, which I delineated in Chapter 1; (2) contemporary structural or "classical" theories that claim they are closest to Freud's position; (3) theories of treatment derived from a consideration of object relations,[1] the present work representing one such example, self psychology another. These different theories reflect disagreements concerning the etiology of the neuroses and therefore propose conflicting treatment goals. Although all psychoanalytic theories include the fundamental elements of the therapeutic process—transference, resistance, and interpretation—the meaning of these terms varies within the context of a given theory.

Freud's theory of therapeutic action, as discussed earlier, does not recognize the significance of the analytic relationship; "classical" theory continues to believe that the insight that results from interpretation is the principal means through which therapeutic change is effected (Valenstein 1979);[2] self psychology focuses upon one mode of object-relatedness (the self and selfobject) to the exclusion of others and ignores or minimizes the function of transference repetition and transference interpretation. These and other issues will be examined in greater detail in this chapter.

One must recognize, however, that the attempt to classify contemporary theories of psychoanalytic treatment leads to little more than convenient fictions. Psychoanalytic theories of treatment are like political parties, where the manifest credo covers very disparate beliefs. For it is difficult, in many instances, to place individual analysts beneath these arbitrary headings. Mitchell (1988), in discussing theories of therapeutic action, was aware of this difficulty; nevertheless he divided theories of treatment as follows: (1) the *drive-conflict model,* which characterizes Freud's theory of treatment; (2) a *developmental arrest model,* which Mitchell associates with the contributions of Winnicott and Kohut; (3) a *relational-conflict model,* which places emphasis on the internal representation of the object rather than upon the (external) object itself.

Pine (1988) also described multiple theories of therapeutic action divided along similar lines: these are theories derived from the psychologies of *drive, ego, object relations,* and *self.* Pine believes, as I do, that the meaning of each therapeutic element, such as interpretation, resistance, and transference, is altered in accordance with the given theoretical context in which such terms appear.

These differences among psychoanalytic theories of treatment become clearer when they are viewed from a historical perspective. For example, the controversy regarding transference gratification, which is linked to the further question of whether the aim of treatment is insight or a corrective emotional experience, can be traced to the historic dispute that occurred between Freud and Ferenczi in the early 1930s. The details of this quarrel are now better known to us through the publication of the *Clinical Diary of Sándor Ferenczi* (Ferenczi 1988) and will be further amplified when the Freud-Ferenczi correspondence is translated into English.[3]

The Freud-Ferenczi Controversy

Freud's theory of treatment can be found, for the most part, in his papers on technique. He broadened the concept of resistance in "Inhibitions, Symptoms and Anxiety," but otherwise, as I have noted, he did not add anything of significance to the theory of treatment. His papers on technique were intended to be primarily an instruction manual for physicians, an attempt to combat the spread of "wild" analysis. The supposition that the theory of the therapeutic action of psychoanalysis was a subject that did not particularly interest Freud is reinforced by the Freud-Ferenczi correspondence. The following is Ferenczi's reply, dated January 17, 1930, to a letter of Freud's (quoted by J. Dupont in Ferenczi 1988, Introduction, p. xiii):⁻

> I do not share, for instance, your view that the therapeutic process is negligible or unimportant, and that simply because it appears less interesting to us, we should ignore it. I, too, have often felt "fed up"[4] in this respect, but overcame this tendency, and I am glad to inform you that precisely in this area a whole series of questions have now come into a new, a sharper focus, perhaps even the problem of repression.

Ferenczi's most important difference with Freud was his belief that the neuroses were largely traumatic in their origin; in this he revived a theory that Freud had abandoned. Ferenczi believed that Freud may have overestimated the role of fantasy and underestimated the role of actual trauma that occurs in parent-child interactions. Ferenczi was thinking not only of sexual seduction of the child by an adult but also of the trauma that results from parental hypocrisy, that is, from a false *affective* relationship with a parent. He foresaw that parental inauthenticity and insensitivity regarding the child's personhood would have profound consequences for the child's sense of self and his relation to reality. In this he anticipates the later contributions of Winnicott and Kohut. This developmental trauma, Ferenczi believed, would be reinforced by the analyst's professional hypocrisy and technical rigidity (Ferenczi 1988). Because of these convictions, Ferenczi believed that psychoanalytic treatment should attempt to restore a "kind, understanding and enlightening environment" (p. 210). Ferenczi was, in this respect, the predecessor of analysts such as Balint, Winnicott, and Loewald who believed that psychoanalytic treatment represents a "new" object relationship and a new beginning.

Inasmuch as Ferenczi believed that his patients had been traumatized, this "new" psychoanalytic relationship represented an attempt to restore or compensate for that which had been absent in the parent-child interaction. Therefore, in contrast to Freud's theory of therapeutic action, Ferenczi believed that the psychoanalytic relationship was a means of ameliorating traumatic experiences. From there it was a short step to claiming that the transference recreated a mother-child relationship in which developmental conflicts could be symbolically actualized, as I have suggested, or that the transference regressively recreated very early developmental stages, as Balint and Winnicott proposed. Ferenczi began to experiment with his "active" treatment, which Freud objected to because he believed that Ferenczi's attempt to cure his patients by means of love would ultimately lead Ferenczi onto the path of sexual seduction.

It is evident that the Freud-Ferenczi controversy continues today between those analysts who emphasize the contribution of the environment in the etiology of the neuroses and hence view psychoanalytic treatment as restorative, and those who emphasize the intrapsychic origin of the neuroses (allowing, of course, for constitutional factors) and are critical of psychoanalytic procedures that are judged to be gratifying. This distrust leads some analysts to condemn object-relations theory, which they believe supports an excessive gratification of the patient by means of the transference. For example, Friedman (1978) reviewed the symposium on "The Curative Factors in Psychoanalysis" that took place at the International Psychoanalytic Congress in Edinburgh in 1961. He considered particularly the controversy that followed Gitelson's (1962) attribution of the curative effect of psychoanalysis to an open dyadic system reminiscent of a mother-child relationship. The opposition replied that only understanding (from interpretation) was curative. Friedman then adds his own comment that "object-relations theory was an attempt to resolve this problem but the destruction it wrought in the theory of the mind discouraged some analysts from pursuing the line of thought" (1978, p. 564).

In a famous letter to Ferenczi (quoted in Gay 1988, p. 578) Freud states: "You have made no secret of the fact that you kiss your patients and let them kiss you. To be sure a kiss may be perceived as harmless. People in the Soviet Union were very free with such salutations. But that does not alter the fact that we are not living in Russia and that with us a kiss signifies an unmistakable erotic intimacy." It is somewhat ironic that Ferenczi, in his *Clinical Diary*, explains that the kissing to which Freud objected resulted from his giving up his "active" treatment in favor of a more passive approach (1988, p. 94). It was this passive experiment that led to the difficulty. The diary reveals (p. 2) that a patient (identified as the American analyst Clara Mabel Thompson) "complied" with Ferenczi's passivity and allowed herself to take the liberty of kissing him. She later boasted to others that "I am allowed to kiss Papa Ferenczi as often as I like."

Ferenczi's egalitarian, nonhypocritical attitude led to an experiment in mutual analysis in which he and the patient alternately exchanged roles as the analyst. Ferenczi experimented in this fashion with two patients but gave it up for a multitude of reasons, not the least of which was the fact that he was placing at risk the confidentiality of his other analytic relationships. Although this experiment now strikes us as naive and imprudent, Ferenczi was struggling with therapeutic dilemmas that are still very much with us. For example, Ferenczi was confronted with the problem that it was hypocritical to withhold information regarding a negative countertransference; psychoanalysts had not yet discovered how a negative countertransference could be placed at the service of the patient's treatment. One of the patients with whom he experimented was someone whom he disliked but who, at the same time, had the transference illusion that Ferenczi was in love with her. By means of this mutual analysis Ferenczi was able to reveal to this patient certain antipathetic countertransference attitudes that were hindering the progress of the treatment, and following his confession, the treatment did in fact move forward.

The matter of equality between analyst and analysand is still a current therapeutic issue. As I discussed earlier, this dilemma reflects the presence of two different levels of reality: the necessary inequality within the frame, which coexists with the equality outside of the frame. Echoes of Ferenczi's egalitarian concerns can be heard in Kohut's advice that the analyst acknowledge his own empathic failures, and Gill's objection to the concept that transference distorts, which assumes that it is the *analyst* who is the judge of what is real.

Freud and Object-Relations Theory

The concept of the psychoanalytic setting is derived directly from object-relations theory (Modell 1988b). Inasmuch as what is now known as object-relations theory was not part of Freud's intellectual assumptions, Freud omitted consideration of the psychoanalytic setting, or gave it only passing notice as the unobjectionable positive transference. This omission may have been reinforced by the composition of Freud's analytic practice. If Freud had been confronted with a series of patients for whom the analytic relationship itself was problematic, he could not have taken this relationship for granted.

Although Freud recognized after the "Project for a Scientific Psychology" that psychoanalysis stood on its own feet and was not a psychological neurology, he never wavered in his belief that important elements of psychoanalytic theory must be supported by evolutionary biology. Freud's belief in the Oedipus complex and his psychosexual theory of development were buttressed by his assumption that the Oedipus complex was consistent with evolutionary biology. Apart from Darwin's publication of *The Expression of Emotion in Man and Animals* in 1872, there were no studies of the evolution of behavior until Lorenz in 1927 and subsequently Tinbergen introduced the science now known as ethology (Mayr 1982). For it is from ethological investigations that we now recognize the universality of "attachment behavior" (in mammals). Freud therefore had no reason to believe that object-relatedness had evolutionary significance. In "Three Essays on Sexuality" (1905a, p. 181) Freud viewed the mother's life-preservative function with regard to her infant to be primarily that of feeding: "The satisfaction of the erotogenic zone is associated, in the first instance, with the satisfaction of the need for nourishment. To begin with, sexuality attaches itself to functions serving the purpose of self-preservation and does not become independent of them until later."

As Laplanche and Pontalis (1973) indicate, the object in Freud's original conception has no conditions imposed upon it other than the requirement that it produce satisfaction. Objects in the oral stage were interchangeable: the term *object* was not equivalent to a person. Thus the idea of an object relationship played no part in Freud's earlier theory. Freud also believed in primary narcissism, that following birth the young infant was self-absorbed and not in a state of object-relatedness with its mother—a view that is thoroughly discredited by observation of infants. This led Winnicott to comment that "in one sense Freud can be said to have neglected infancy as a state" (1965, p. 39). It was not until the last decades of his life, coincident with the development of structural theory, that Freud focused his attention upon object relationships and underlined the importance of the loss of the object. In a certain sense the vicissitudes of object attachment and loss can be said to be at the center of structural theory, which is a theory of the internalization that follows the loss of the object (Freud 1923a, p. 29): "the character of the ego is a precipitate of abandoned object-cathexes and . . . it contains the history of those object choices."

In "Inhibitions, Symptoms and Anxiety" (1926) Freud emphasized the importance of object loss in symptom formation and thereby acknowledged the importance of dependency. He explained that the child's safety in the world depended upon the presence of a protective object, and that the loss or threat of loss of this object resulted in a stereotypical response of anxiety analogous to those instinctive responses noted in other species. The human child depends upon its caretakers to provide those signals of danger that are the instinctive endowment of other species (1926, p. 168): "Man seems not to have been endowed, or to have been endowed to only a very small degree, with an instinctive recognition of the dangers that threaten him from without. Small children are constantly doing things which endanger their lives, and that is precisely why they cannot afford to be without a protecting object."

It was Bowlby (1969) who marshaled the evidence that demonstrated the close analogy between attachment behavior in primates and the object relationship between mother and child. He drew the important conclusion that attachment behavior and sexuality represent two separate organizing systems within the personality.[5] Bowlby demonstrated that the mother's love and presence are as important to the young child's survival as is the provision of food. Whatever name we choose to call the "instinct" that underlies attachment behavior, it is something apart from the tension reduction or orgastic release that characterizes sexuality. Winnicott (1965), who was a colleague of Bowlby's, also contrasted what he called *ego-relatedness* with the tension reduction that accompanies nursing, describing some mothers who, instead of relating to their infants, "fob them off" with a feed.

What Bowlby described as attachment behavior becomes the underlying matrix of the psychoanalytic setting. The psychoanalytic setting functions as a protective environment interposed between the self and the real world. It creates, in Sandler's (1960) term, a "background of safety." *This object tie to the analyst or therapist is the glue that holds together the entire therapeutic enterprise.*

The Prerequisites of Safety

What one judges to be the conditions of safety in the treatment setup depends upon one's view of the source of danger, which will differ between those who assume a traumatic etiology of the neuroses and those who emphasize intrapsychic (or intrasystemic) conflict. If the etiology of the neuroses is seen as primarily intrapsychic, the source of danger is understood to be that of heightened instinctual tension, which includes the internal persecution of a harsh superego.[6] Safety then is achieved primarily by means of interpretations that extend the domain of the ego's rational control over the irrational internal world of the id, as in Freud's famous aphorism: "where id was there shall ego be" (1933, p. 80). This view of psychoanalytic treatment, characteristic of Freud's earlier period, sees danger in the return of the warded-off contents of the mind that are held in repression by a weakened or compromised ego. Danger consists in pathogenic fantasies, so that interpretations that exorcise these fantasies promote the conditions of safety. Safety is achieved not only by means of interpretation but by the alliance that Freud spoke of between the analyst and analysand against the common enemy—the instinctual demands of the id and the conscientious demands of the superego (Freud 1940). This belief in the power of the analyst's interpretation to remove pathogenic contents finds its clearest expression in Kleinian analysis, which has been characterized by Schafer (1985) as a belief in the omnipotence of interpretation. Glover (1931) also professed a belief in the power of the exact interpretation to free the mind of pathogenic contents.

There is a popular misconception that psychoanalytic treatment regularly results in the recovery of repressed memories. Indeed, some patients fear analysis because they feel that it may uncover some terrible secret that they have repressed and of which they have no awareness. Most analyses do not result in the uncovering of such repressed memories; what *is* recovered, however, is the warded-off affects associated with traumatic experiences. Such affects are reexperienced when the ambience is safe enough to allow for their emergence.[7] That is to say, warded-off affects can materialize without interpretation.[8] Weiss and Sampson (1986) have interpreted the experience of "crying at a happy ending" as evidence that an individual may unconsciously "lift his own defense" and bring forth warded-off content (and affects) when he or she perceives that it is safe enough to do so. This process can be observed in those patients who lost a parent when they were children, and because of their immaturity were unable to complete the work of mourning. When such patients perceive that the psychoanalytic setting is a safe environment, they will permit themselves to complete the work of mourning that was interrupted in childhood.

In order to have a childhood, and not be forced into a precocious maturity, the child must have caretakers who provide an environment that stands between her and the dangers of the real world. Where there are massive failures in this protective parental holding environ-

aspect of the self experience is most evident when there is in the transference and countertransference a recreation of the dissociated and disclaimed parts of the self. In such cases the safety of the psychoanalytic setting will be tested by an unconscious manipulation of the countertransference. Thus psychoanalysis, as a restorative process of the self, must also involve repetition and retranscription.

Winnicott did not refer directly to transference repetition, but it is implicit in his concept of regression to dependency (1965, p. 258):

> So in the end we succeed by failing—failing the patient's way. This is a long distance from the simple theory of cure by corrective experience. In this way, regression can be in the service of the ego if it is met by the analyst, and turned into a new dependence in which the patient brings the bad external factor into the area of his or her omnipotent control . . . the operative factor is that the patient now hates the analyst for the failure that originally came as an environmental factor, outside the infant's area of omnipotent control, but that is *now* staged in the transference.

Interpersonal theorists also avoid the concept of repetition. For example, Levenson (1988), instead of transference repetition, refers to the "recursive order of transference." As I understand the term *recursive,* it denotes variations of nesting such as stories within stories, Russian dolls inside of Russian dolls, and so forth.[11] This is an interesting idea as applied to transference, but it is something different from transference repetition. Gill (1982), who has become an interpersonal theorist, has also de-emphasized the therapeutic value of transference repetition in favor of the "here and now."[12]

What I have objected to in Freud's theory of the repetition compulsion is not that it rests upon certain biological assumptions but that those assumptions are clearly antiquated. Therefore, I found a welcome affirmation of the biological significance of the process of repetition in Gerald Edelman's *Neural Darwinism.* As discussed earlier, Edelman's theory of memory posits that memory does not consist of a permanent record in the brain that is isomorphic with past experience; instead, memory is a dynamic retranscription that is context-bound and established by means of categories. This description of memory is relevant for psychoanalysis in that it accounts for the fact that repetition can lead to novel configurations, an idea that Freud anticipated in his concept of *Nachträglichkeit.* Edelman also emphasized that motoric action is essential for perception. The repetition of affect categories within the transference and countertransference, a form of motor action, acts synergistically with the perceptual system in order to test the safety of the human environment. Perception activates categorical affective memory, which in turn colors current experience. It is this process that psychoanalysis facilitates by means of the multiple realities of the psychoanalytic setting. Through interpretation and symbolic actualization, it is possible to retranscribe time in order to rid oneself of the "tyranny of the past."

Notes

References

Index

Notes

1. Freud's Theory of Psychoanalytic Treatment

1. Thomä believes that Strachey's translation was mistakenly tied to the model of abreaction. Thomä (1989) also notes that Strachey translated *nachträglich* and *Nachträglichkeit* in different ways. I am also indebted to Donald Gerard (personal communication) for his clarification of the term, which he believes in the interest of accuracy should be referred to as *wirken nachträglich*. For a further commentary on Freud's use of the term *nachträglich*, see Laplanche and Pontalis (1973). They note that it is not experience in general that is revised but only what is unassimilated, that is to say, experience that is traumatic (p. 112). As will be seen in later chapters, I may have interpreted Freud's term *nachträglich* more broadly than Freud had intended.

2. Thomä (1989, p. 8) shows how Strachey's translation, *deferred action*, conveys the opposite of what Freud intended: "The primary difference between *nachtragen* and defer consists in the fact that they express exactly opposite relations to time. Both words have the same root, the Latin root being *ferre* which means carry or *tragen*. There is thus an etymological connection with *Übertragung* (transference) and with the word *metaferein*, the Greek verb related to the noun metaphor, whose original meaning was to carry something from here to there and to transfer or extend to another place or later time. And in fact the metaphorical meaning of *nachtragen* (to hold a grudge) is still associated with the word *Nachträglichkeit*. This is lost in English where the verb to grudge is not associated with the verb carry."

3. Weiss and Sampson (1986) distinguish pathogenic beliefs from fantasies in their feeling that beliefs, in contrast to fantasies, are not wishful but grim and constricting. They believe then that therapeutic change results from the disconfirmation of pathogenic beliefs.

4. Ferenczi (1909), much later, rediscovered the resemblance between the hypnotic condition and a parental transference.

5. Jones also adds that this second honeymoon resulted in the conception of a daughter. However, Ellenberger's researches (1970) cast doubt upon this detail of Jones's account.

6. In Breuer's own account of this treatment some twenty-five years later in 1907 (Cranefield 1958), he was careful to differentiate his method of treatment from that of Freud, calling it *analysis* rather than *psychoanalysis*. Freud also in his Encyclopaedia Article (Freud 1923) distinguishes his technique from that

of Breuer, noting that he, in contrast to Breuer, recognized the importance of defense.

7. Ludwig Wittgenstein (1984, p. 36e) offers this comment concerning the relation between Freud's originality and the seed of psychoanalysis introduced by Breuer: "I believe that my originality (if that is the right word) is an originality belonging to the soil rather than to the seed. (Perhaps I have no seed of my own.) Sow a seed in my soil and it will grow differently than it would in any other soil. Freud's originality too was like this, I think. I have always believed—without knowing why—that the real germ of psycho-analysis came from Breuer, not Freud. Of course Breuer's seed-grain can only have been quite tiny. *Courage* is always original."

8. This theory of memory as successive retranscriptions is at odds with Freud's belief in a system of fixed memory that he described elsewhere (*The Interpretation of Dreams*, 1900, and the "Mystic Writing-Pad," 1925). Freud there attributed to mental apparatus two separate systems for the registration of memories: there is a perceptual system (Pcpt.-Cs) which perceives perceptions but retains no permanent traces of them, while the permanent traces of the excitations are preserved in "mnemic systems" lying beyond the perceptual system.

9. Milan Kundera (1984) says in *The Unbearable Lightness of Being* that once is nothing.

10. In the case of the Wolf Man (Freud 1918, p. 44) Freud indicates that the primal scene that was observed at age one and a half was activated, as though it were a recent experience, at age four. In a footnote (p. 103) Freud refers to " 'retrospective phantasying' of late impressions into childhood and their sexualization after the event."

11. This is in contrast to psychoanalysis outside of the United States, especially in France, where, because of the influence of Lacan, the concept of *Nachträglichkeit* has received wide acceptance. As Baranger et al. (1983) observe, if one assimilates this idea one can no longer believe in a strictly linear developmental psychology. They believe that full acceptance of the idea of *Nachträglichkeit* would invalidate developmental theories such as those of Melanie Klein that emphasize the primacy of the earliest experiences, and that this fact has prejudiced analysts against the concept of *Nachträglichkeit*.

12. It is not possible for me to present here an adequate summary of Edelman's difficult but rewarding book. The interested reader should consult Edelman's *Neural Darwinism* (1987) or a commentary on this work by Rosenfeld (1988).

2. Play, Illusion, and the Setting of Psychoanalysis

1. My view, which will be illustrated throughout this work, is that there are fundamental elements in the therapeutic encounter that transcend the differences between psychotherapy and psychoanalysis. My clinical experience derives for the most part from psychoanalysis, which, because of its greater intensity and continuity as compared to psychotherapy, may teach us more about the forces of therapeutic change. This does not mean that one can disregard the differences between psychotherapy and psychoanalysis. The differences in the physical setup, such as the use of the couch and the fact that the analysand does not see the

analyst's face, and the greater frequency of sessions all have significant consequences. Further, it is unquestionably true that there are certain patients who can *only* be treated successfully with psychoanalysis, while there are others for whom psychotherapy is the treatment of choice and for whom psychoanalysis may be contraindicated. But it must also be admitted that a clear statement of the fundamental differences and similarities between psychoanalysis and psychotherapy has continued to elude us. For these reasons I will not always differentiate the terms *therapist* and *analyst*.

2. The existence of multiple realities and paradox in the therapeutic setting was observed in psychotic patients by Kafka (1964), who noted its implication for psychoanalysis.

3. London (1987) also used this example of Huizinga's to illustrate the illusion of transference. Although London's point of view is similar to my own, he would restrict the playful or ludic aspects of transference to the transference neurosis and describes other forms of transference as nonludic. As I shall discuss in a later section, this restricted view of transference cannot be supported.

4. Ogden (1985) describes Winnicott's potential space as a dialectic between fantasy and reality.

5. The application of "frame" theory to the psychoanalytic interaction was reviewed by Vann Spruiell (1983), who also emphasized the significance of the "rules of the game."

6. Hearne tells how one communicates to dogs: when you say something you must really mean it. As in psychoanalysis, there is no room for inauthenticity.

7. For example, Lacan (1978) observed that it is the analyst who directs the treatment, and it is the analyst who is the one who *knows*.

8. False or exaggerated affects may be used in the service of a defense against communication. Since genuine communication is object-seeking, spurious affects create distance. Further, exaggeratedly intense or overly dramatic affects may be used to create a sense of "aliveness" when what is feared is psychic deadness (Modell 1984a).

9. For an extensive discussion of Freud's views on the reality of dreams, see O'Flaherty (1984).

10. Psychoanalytic observations of schizophrenic patients, who are in touch with the deepest meaning of their experiences, offer us clues to processes that are otherwise obscured in the healthier patient. Arvanitakis (1987) observed that for the schizophrenic the frame of the treatment may be experienced as a primitive body image, a body image shared between therapist and patient.

11. Margaret Little (1985), in her autobiographical account of her analysis with Winnicott, reveals that she was the patient that Winnicott described in this quote. She relates that she was seized with recurring spasms of terror which built up throughout her entire body, reached a climax, and subsided. When this occurred in an analytic session, she grabbed Winnicott's hands and clung tightly until the spasm passed: "He said that he thought that she was reliving the experience of being born: He held my head for a few minutes, saying that immediately after birth an infant's head could ache and feel heavy for a time." Little confirms my assertion that for Winnicott regression was both literal and metaphoric.

12. See also Modell (1976).

13. For further discussion of Winnicott's concept of regression, see Modell (1985a).

14. In this chapter I have been describing the therapeutic or beneficial effects of dependency when the analytic setting is experienced as a holding environment. It should be noted, however, that a very different position concerning the uses of dependency was voiced by Macalpine (1950), who suggests that the analyst forces the patient into an undesirable childlike role. Macalpine believed that in the analyst's attempt to maintain the "purity" of the analytic situation, the analyst "induced" a regressive transference. She attributed this "induced" regression to a combination of many factors, including that of sensory deprivation—the prohibition of looking at the analyst. Where I have described elements of the analytic setting as contributing to the analysand's sense of safety and being held, Macalpine saw these same elements as infantilizing. She asserted that the analyst's constancy was experienced by the analysand as a "strict infantile routine." She believed that the analysand was further infantilized by the analyst's silence and his or her failure to respond to questions; in her opinion this leads to diminished personal responsibility and induction of magical expectations, which is an expression of the overwhelming authority of the analyst. The analysand, according to Macalpine, has no recourse but to adapt to this infantilizing environment by a "regression."

15. There are, of course, many evident differences between parental care and the analytic setting, which need not be enumerated.

16. This Jacksonian schema of the central nervous system continues to have a pervasive, if perhaps unrecognized, influence on contemporary psychoanalytic thinking. For example, Gedo and Goldberg's *Models of the Mind* (1973) views the mind as a similar hierarchically organized system, starting from the most primitive reflex-arc model of automatic response and ending with a mode of functioning that is volitional and complex.

17. Gould (1977, p. 96) notes that belief in Haeckel's law was combined frequently with a neo-Lamarckianism in which there is an analogy made between the intensity of memory and heredity: "Instincts are the unconscious remembrance of things learned so strongly, impressed so indelibly into memory, that the germ cells are affected and pass the trait to future generations."

3. *Transference and Levels of Reality*

1. The psychoanalytic setting has also been referred to as the "non-process" background that contains the "process" (Baranger et al., 1983).

2. For reasons different from my own, Gill (1982) has also objected to the distinction these authors have made between the "real" relationship and transference, and to the use of the term "distortion of reality." Gill suggests that a consensually validated concept of the actual situation be "negotiated" between the two participants. Schwaber (1983) has also emphasized that the analyst's reality is not necessarily the patient's reality.

3. Wollheim (1984) also used the term *iconic* to refer to mental events. Although the word is commonly applied to visual images, it can be used to denote a

specificity and particularity. Wollheim stated (1984, p. 62): "In the first place, iconic mental states may be of mere individuals, but standardly they are of events. These events contain their own characters, and these characters constitute the dramatis personae . . . parents, lovers, historical figures . . . Iconic mental states regularly occur in sequences and, as the states succeed one another, so the dramatis personae interact, the events make up a story, a narrative unfolds."

4. Friedman (1969) claims that Freud resolved the paradox that transference is both the motor of cure and the major obstacle to cure by distinguishing the transference neurosis from the unobjectionable positive transference. I believe that this distinction refers to categories of transference, not the paradox of transference.

5. What is recreated here confirms Fairbairn's important observation (1952) that the schizoid patient feels that her love is dangerous and "bad."

6. Zetzel (1956) criticized the logic of Melanie Klein's theories because of a confusion of fantasy and process.

7. Projective identification has also been interpreted as something analogous to Anna Freud's concept of identification with the aggressor (Porder 1987). Although role reversals of this sort can be often observed (as in my cases), I believe that to attempt to place this phenomenon within the more familiar category of defenses of the ego ignores Bion's important observation that projective identification is a form of communication.

4. Repetition and Retranscription

1. For further discussion of this point see Rosenfeld (1988).

2. Freud distinguished affects and ideation (1915, p. 178): ". . . but in comparison with unconscious ideas there is the important difference that unconscious ideas continue to exist after repression as actual structures in the system *Ucs.*, whereas all that corresponds in that system to unconscious affects is a potential beginning which is prevented from developing."

3. Green (1975) has also noted that affects are never without semantic content.

4. Freud (1909, p. 208n.) illustrated in the case of the Rat Man that the Oedipus complex, which he called the *nuclear complex of the neuroses,* consists largely of biologically rooted fantasies: "The uniformity of the contents of the sexual life of children . . . will easily account for the constant sameness which as a rule characterizes the phantasies that are constructed around the period of childhood, irrespective of how greatly or how little real experiences have contributed towards them." In the case of the Wolf Man, Freud also described the Oedipus complex as experience remodeled by the phylogenetic schemata (primal fantasies) (1918, p. 118).

5. See Modell (1984a) for further discussion of this point.

6. Kohut, who has minimized man's darker destructive nature, has not sufficiently recognized that the idealized self may represent a split-off portion of the hated self. However, he did appreciate the defensive function of the grandiosity that accompanies such idealizations.

7. Alexander and French describe the analyst's manipulation of the treatment

as the "Principle of Flexibility." For example, "When the intensity of . . . hostile impulses is too low, it may be well to let it increase by lessening the frequency of interviews" (1946, p. 30).

8. In this respect I disagree with Kohut (1984), who has tended to view the patient as a passive partner in the therapeutic interaction. For example, Kohut suggests that the therapist should apologize for his failure to understand the patient. No doubt, at times, the therapist is responsible for misunderstanding his patient; but I believe that more often it is the patient who controls our access to understanding. The therapist's misunderstanding frequently represents the recreation of a specific absence, that is to say, an attempt to bring what was experienced passively into one's active control.

5. Experiencing Time

1. Namnum (1972) describes the psychoanalytic setup as designed in part as a manipulation of the experience of time, in that the analytic procedure is thought to be timeless yet the analysand is confronted with a rigidity and control of the arrangements of present time. This juxtaposition of timelessness and inflexibility regarding the arrangements of current time, he believes, promotes the experience of time past.

2. The practice of Zen Buddhism, while not at all related to the manic defense, achieves something similar by very different means.

3. Bergler and Roheim (1946) suggest that the passage of time symbolizes separation; timelessness is the fantasy in which mother and child are endlessly united.

4. Kafka (1977) has said that the analyst is both a "condenser" and "dilator" of time.

5. Rosenfeld (1988) also uses Proust to illustrate that *memory without the present cannot exist.*

6. Gross (1949) believed that references to time in dreams pertain to *current* object relationships.

7. Michael Sherwood (1969) offered an extensive gloss on Freud's case history of the Rat Man, from which he concluded that Freud's account was essentially a narrative explanation and not something that is in accord with a scientific hypothetical-deductive mode of thought.

8. I have made my own position on this matter clear elsewhere (Modell 1984a); I prefer to think that the existence of the scientific and hermeneutic constructions of reality is a paradox that we should not attempt to resolve.

6. The Act of Interpretation

1. Freud admits: "I did not succeed in mastering the transference in good time . . . I neglected the precaution of looking out for the first signs of transference . . . At the beginning it was clear that I was replacing her father in her imagination" (1905, p. 118).

2. I have placed quotation marks around the expression "giving" or "making"

interpretations, for such terms are misleading in that an interpretation is likened to a procedure attributable to the analyst alone.

3. Wolff (1988) offers the radical proposal that the differentiation between historical truth and narrative truth is irrelevant (1988, p. 404) in that: "personal desire and its disguised expressions are constantly shaped by the experience of history and that our experience of history is constantly determined by our personal desire, both dimensions being part of one coherent psycho-biography that cannot be arbitrarily divided into historical and narrative truth."

4. For further discussion of constructivist philosophy and its influence on psychology, see Watzlawick (1984) and Bruner (1986).

5. I described a case (Modell 1985) where, because of the unreliability of the parental holding environment, learning from others was nearly totally precluded.

6. The use of the analyst as a "prosthesis" is most evident in those cases where there is a cognitive deficit. Such a case was described by Gedo (1984), where the patient, a psychologist, lacked the capacity for empathy and made use of the analyst's empathy as if it were a tool or a prosthesis. Gedo (1988) has emphasized the remedial instruction that occurs in the psychoanalytic process in which the analyst is used as a prosthesis.

7. Loewald (1980, p. 238) made essentially the same point: "The higher organizational stage of the environment is indispensable for the development of the psychic apparatus and, in the early stages has to be brought to it actively. Without such a differential between the organism and the environment no development takes place."

8. Freud (1933) rejected a psychoanalytic Weltanschauung because he claimed that psychoanalysis was part of a scientific Weltanschauung.

9. See Pontalis (1981) on the dream as an object.

7. The Schizoid Dilemma

1. For an alternative explanation, see the discussion of affect categories in Chapter 4.

2. For an excellent contemporary view of the various ideas included under the heading of *resistance,* see Thomä and Kächele (1987).

3. For discussion of this point see Modell (1984a).

4. One thinks of Schopenhauer's tale of the freezing porcupines, as quoted by Freud (1921, p. 101): "A company of porcupines crowded themselves very close together on a cold winter's day so as to profit from one another's warmth and to save themselves from being frozen to death. But soon they felt one another's quills, which induced them to separate again, and the second evil arose once more. So that they were driven backwards and forwards from one trouble to the other, until they discovered a mean distance at which they could most tolerably exist."

5. For a more extensive discussion of this point see Modell 1984a.

6. There is accumulating evidence from studies of social evolution of inherent conflict between parents and their offspring because of a genetic divergence (Trivers 1985). From this it can be inferred that the difference between the parent's

construction of reality and the child's construction of reality may reflect this divergence. For the application of this important concept to psychoanalysis, see Slavin (1985).

8. The Patient's Use of the Therapist

1. King (1962, p. 226) said: "I sometimes think of the analytic relationship as a psychological stage on which I as analyst am committed to take whatever role my patient may unconsciously assign to me."

2. For further discussion of knowledge and forms of loving, see Modell (1968).

3. Gedo and Goldberg (1973) have adopted this particular strategy in that they correlate four developmental phases with corresponding therapeutic action: Phase I—pacification; Phase II—unification; Phase III—optimal disillusion; Phase IV—interpretation.

4. I do not believe that there are any fundamental differences in technique in the psychoanalysis of the so-called narcissistic personality disorder as compared to the classical neuroses. It is a matter of the *patient* choosing, during a specific phase of the treatment, to utilize and concentrate upon a given element from the array of therapeutic procedures that are intrinsic to "standard" technique. For example, some patients who need to protect their self-created reality will respond to the analyst's interpretations only as a metacommunication or as a piece of symbolic action and will ignore the ostensive content of the interpretation. As the treatment progresses, interpretations will then be used for their ostensive content.

5. Stern's criticism (1985) of Mahler's developmental theories is consistent with this point of view.

6. Newman (1984) compared Winnicott's "use of the object" to analogous concepts to be found in the contributions of Melanie Klein and Kohut.

7. We know from the biographical accounts that some great artists cannot work without the presence of their muse. For some, creative activity was absolutely contingent on the presence of a woman, who could be interchangeable. One thinks, for example, of Picasso, Robert Graves, and T. S. Eliot. For Eliot, however, his schizophrenic wife, Vivienne, proved to be a negative muse who contributed to the pain that he transmuted into poetry; his survival depended upon a loving muse, Emily Hale, although he eventually found her to be dispensable (Gordon 1988).

8. Coleridge viewed the act of knowing as a "coalescence of the Subject and the Object . . . the self has gone into what it perceives, and what it perceives is in this sense itself" (quoted in I. A. Richards 1969). Coleridge may have been the first to appreciate the acquisition of knowledge through the play of merging and separateness.

9. For a review of this topic see Meissner (1988).

10. For a review of the concepts of the therapeutic and working alliance see Thomä and Kächele (1986).

11. I would agree with Brenner that the therapeutic alliance is subject to a symbolic transformation and cannot be excluded from the category of transfer-

ence. However, this is true of nearly all human behavior. But Brenner is mistaken in failing to recognize that the therapeutic alliance is a phenomenon that is quite different from the transference neurosis. (For a more complete discussion see Chapters 2 and 3.)

9. Paradox and Therapeutic Dilemmas

1. For a discussion of this issue see Watzlawick, Bavelas, and Jackson (1967).

2. I owe this particular example to Watzlawick, Bavelas, and Jackson (1967).

3. Anton Kris (1977) considered either-or dilemmas as conflicts in which the *patient* assumes there can be no resolution. Kris would later make a distinction between *convergent* and *divergent* conflicts (Kris 1985). I believe that Kris's observations also have their origin in the fundamentally paradoxical nature of the self.

4. For further discussion of this issue see Wallerstein (1983), Treurniet (1980), and Modell (1984b).

5. This quest for self-actualization and autonomy may reflect a search for hopefulness not in relationship to the world, where one is powerless, but in the hope of modifying the self (Morgenthau and Person 1978).

6. Ferenczi was also aware of this paradox, as I shall describe in the next chapter. His failed experiment in mutual analysis was an attempt to establish a state of equality between analyst and analysand.

7. Parsons (1986) interprets Bion's aphorism to mean that the analyst should maintain a state of non-attachment regarding her *understanding* of the analysand.

8. When I began my psychoanalytic training in the 1950s one heard stories, possibly apocryphal, of analysts who remained silent even when the analysand said "Hello." Some analysts became a caricature of themselves for fear of doing anything that might interfere with the development of the transference. This led to a style of practicing psychoanalysis that could, charitably, be called austere abstinence. Leo Stone's (1961) important contribution was in part a reaction against this mistaken adherence to Freud's "principle" of abstinence. Stone reminded his audience that the dependent physician-like relationship of which psychoanalysis was one example provided legitimate forms of gratification.

9. Freud later explained (1919, p. 163) that treatment should occur in a state of abstinence because gratification may remove the symptoms prematurely, and the analysand would then lose his motivation to continue the treatment.

10. Gedo (1988) uses the term *enactment* in a similar fashion.

10. Theories of Psychoanalytic Treatment

1. One must also recognize the diversity of object-relations theories. Indeed, there is an important distinction between the contributions of Melanie Klein and Fairbairn, who have placed such emphasis upon the internal object, and the theories of those such as Balint, Winnicott, and myself, who have emphasized the external object. However, it now appears that this distinction may become less

relevant since contemporary Kleinians stress, above all, the importance of projective identification, a process that encompasses both internal and external object relations.

2. This statement is frequently accompanied by a disparagement of corrective emotional experiences. Valenstein (1979) refers to "interpersonally promoted experiential effects leading to transference 'cures.' "

3. For a recent account of this controversy between Freud and Ferenczi, see Gedo (1986).

4. Ferenczi refers in his Journal to a remark that "Freud let fall in my presence, obviously relying on my discretion: 'Patients are a rabble' " (1988, p. 93).

5. I have suggested elsewhere (Modell 1975, 1984a, 1985b) that the distinction between attachment behavior and sexuality is consistent with Freud's earlier distinction between the "ego instincts" or the instinct for self-preservation and the sexual instincts, a classification proposed as an interim hypothesis prior to Freud's introduction of the death instinct.

6. Freud viewed the superego's persecution of the ego (or self) as a manifestation of the id (1923a, p. 36): "By setting up this ego ideal, the ego has mastered the Oedipus complex and at the same time placed itself in subjection to the id. Whereas the ego is essentially the representative of the external world, of reality, the super-ego stands in contrast to it as the representative of the internal world, of the id."

7. An exception to this statement would be the automatic repetition of affect categories, as in projective identification. Such repetition does not require the perception of a safe environment. However, the compulsive repetition of affect categories can be understood as a sampling of the environment in order to test the conditions of safety. As described in the previous chapter, it may be necessary, paradoxically, to first create a situation of danger in order to reassure oneself that it is safe.

8. See also Eagle's preface to Weiss and Sampson (1986).

9. For further discussion of this observation see Modell (1988a).

10. There is nothing to suggest, however, that Ferenczi depreciated the importance of transference repetition.

11. For a lively account of recursion see Hofstadter (1979).

12. Stone (1981) reviewed Gill's theory of the "here and now" from a historical perspective.

References

Alexander, F., and T. French. 1946. *Psycho-analytic Therapy.* New York: Ronald Press.

Anzieu, D. 1986. Paradoxical transference. *Contemporary Psychoanalysis* 22:520–547.

Arlow, J. 1959. The structure of the déjà-vu experience. *Journal of the American Psychoanalytic Association* 7:611–631.

——— 1984. Disturbances of the sense of time: With special reference to the experience of timelessness. *Psychoanalytic Quarterly* 53:13–37.

——— 1986. Psychoanalysis and time. *Journal of the American Psychoanalytic Association* 34:507–528.

Arvanitakis, K. 1987. The analytic frame in the treatment of schizophrenia and its relation to depression. *International Journal of Psycho-analysis* 68:525–533.

Augustine, Saint. 397. *Confessions.* London: J. M. Dent, 1939.

Balint, M. 1968. *The Basic Fault.* London: Tavistock Publications.

Baranger, M., et al. 1983. Process and non-process in analytic work. *International Journal of Psycho-analysis* 64:1–15.

Bateson, G. 1972. A theory of play and fantasy. In *Steps to an Ecology of Mind.* New York: Ballantine.

Bergler, E., and G. Roheim. 1946. Psychology of time perception. *Psychoanalytic Quarterly* 15:190–206.

Bibring, E. 1954. Psychoanalysis and the dynamic psychotherapies. *Journal of the American Psychoanalytic Association* 2:745–770.

Bion, W. 1962. Learning from experience. In *Seven Servants.* New York: Jason Aronson.

——— 1970. *Attention and Interpretation.* New York: Basic Books.

Bleger, J. 1967. Psycho-analysis of the psychoanalytic frame. *International Journal of Psycho-analysis* 48:511–519.

Blum, H. 1971. On the conception and development of the transference neurosis. *Journal of the American Psychoanalytic Association* 19:41–53.

Bohr, N. 1958. Light and life. In *Atomic Physics and Human Knowledge*. New York: Wiley.

Bonaparte, M. 1940. Time and the unconscious. *International Journal of Psycho-analysis* 21:427–468.

Bowlby, J. 1969. *Attachment and Loss*. Vol. 1, *Attachment*. New York: Basic Books.

Brenner, C. 1979. Working alliance, therapeutic alliance and transference. *Journal of the American Psychoanalytic Association* 27 (supplement):137–157.

Breuer, J. and S. Freud. 1893. *Studies in Hysteria*. S.E. 2.

Bruner, J. 1985. Vygotsky: A historical and conceptual perspective. In *Culture Communication and Cognition*, ed. J. Wertsch. Cambridge: Cambridge University Press.

———— 1986. *Actual Minds, Possible Worlds*. Cambridge, Mass.: Harvard University Press.

Calvino, I. 1986. *The Uses of Literature*, trans. P. Creagh. New York: Harcourt Brace Jovanovich.

———— 1986a. De Chirico City. *FMR* 4:85–98.

Campbell, J. 1983. *The Way of the Animal Powers*, vol. 1. San Francisco: Alfred Van Der Marck Editions.

Chertok, L., and de Saussure, R. 1979. *The Therapeutic Revolution: From Mesmer to Freud*. New York: Brunner/Mazel.

Cooper, A. 1987. The transference neurosis: A concept ready for retirement. *Psychoanalytic Inquiry* 7:569–585.

Cranefield, P. 1958. Joseph Breuer's evaluation of his contribution to psychoanalysis. *International Journal of Psycho-analysis* 39: 319–322.

Draenos, S. 1982. *Freud's Odyssey*. New Haven: Yale University Press.

Eagle, M. 1984. *Recent Developments in Psychoanalysis*. New York: McGraw-Hill.

Edelman, G. 1987. *Neural Darwinism*. New York: Basic Books.

Eliade, M. 1959. *Cosmos and History: The Myth of the Eternal Return*. New York: Harper.

Eliot, T. S. 1962. *The Complete Poems and Plays*. New York: Harcourt, Brace and World.

Ellenberger, H. 1970. *The Discovery of the Unconscious*. New York: Basic Books.

Fairbairn, W. R. D. 1952. *Psychoanalytic Studies of the Personality.* London: Tavistock.

Ferenczi, S. 1909. Introjection and transference. In *Sex and Psychoanalysis.* New York: Brunner, 1950.

———— 1988. *The Clinical Diary of Sándor Ferenczi,* ed. J. Dupont. Cambridge, Mass.: Harvard University Press.

Flavell, J. 1963. *The Developmental Psychology of Jean Piaget.* Princeton, N.J.: Van Nostrand.

Fox, R. 1984. Principle of abstinence reconsidered. *International Review of Psycho-analysis* 11:227–236.

Freud, A. 1936. *The Ego and the Mechanisms of Defense.* New York: International Universities Press.

———— 1969. *Difficulties in the Path of Psychoanalysis.* New York: International Universities Press.

———— 1971. The infantile neurosis: Genetic and dynamic considerations. *Psychoanalytic Study of the Child* 26:79–90.

Freud, S. 1895. Project for a scientific psychology. The Standard Edition of the *Complete Psychological Works of Sigmund Freud,* trans. J. Strachey (hereafter S. E.). London: Hogarth Press, 1966. Vol. 1.

———— 1896. Further remarks on the neuro-psychoses of defense. S. E., vol. 3.

———— 1898. Sexuality in the aetiology of the neuroses. S. E., vol. 3.

———— 1900. *The Interpretation of Dreams.* S. E., vols. 4 and 5.

———— 1901. *The Psychopathology of Everyday Life.* S. E., vol. 6.

———— 1905. Fragment of an analysis of a case of hysteria. S. E., vol. 7.

———— 1905a. Three essays on the theory of sexuality. S. E., vol. 7.

———— 1907. Jensen's gravida. S. E., vol. 9.

———— 1909. Notes upon a case of obsessional neurosis. S. E., vol. 10.

———— 1912. The dynamics of transference. S. E., vol. 12.

———— 1912a. Recommendations to physicians practicing psychoanalysis. S. E., vol. 12.

———— 1914. Remembering, repeating and working-through (Further recommendations on the technique of psychoanalysis, II). S. E., vol. 12.

———— 1915. Observations on transference love (Further recommendations on the technique of psycho-analysis, III). S. E., vol. 12.

———— 1915a. The unconscious. S. E., vol. 14.

———— 1917. Introductory lectures on psychoanalysis (General theory of the neuroses). S. E., vol. 16.

———— 1918. From the history of an infantile neurosis. S. E., vol. 17.

———— 1919. Lines of advance in psycho-analytic therapy. S. E., vol. 17.

———— 1920. The psychogenesis of a case of homosexuality in a woman. S. E., vol. 18.

———— 1920a. Beyond the pleasure principle. S. E., vol. 18.

———— 1921. Group psychology and the analysis of the ego. S. E., vol. 18.

———— 1923. Two encyclopaedia articles. S. E., vol. 18.

———— 1923a. The ego and the id. S. E., vol. 19.

———— 1925. Negation. S. E., vol. 19.

———— 1925a. A note upon the "mystic writing-pad." S. E., vol. 19.

———— 1926. Inhibitions, symptoms and anxiety. S. E., vol. 20.

———— 1933. The new introductory lectures. S. E., vol. 22.

———— 1937. Analysis terminable and interminable. S. E., vol. 23.

———— 1940. An outline of psychoanalysis. S. E., vol. 23.

———— 1987. *A Phylogenetic Fantasy: Overview of the Transference Neuroses,* ed. Ilse Grubrich-Simitis, trans. Axel Hoffer and Peter T. Hoffer. Cambridge, Mass.: Harvard University Press.

Friedman, L. 1969. The therapeutic alliance. *International Journal of Psycho-analysis* 50:139–153.

———— 1978. Trends in the psychoanalytic theory of treatment. *Psychoanalytic Quarterly* 47:524–567.

Gay, P. 1988. *Freud: A Life for Our Time.* New York: Norton.

Gedo, J., and A. Goldberg. 1973. *Models of the Mind.* Chicago: University of Chicago Press.

———— 1984. *Psychoanalysis and Its Discontents.* New York: Guilford Press.

———— 1988. *The Mind in Disorder.* Hillsdale, N.J.: Analytic Press.

Gill, M. 1982. *Analysis of Transference,* vol. 1. New York: International Universities Press.

Gitelson, M. 1962. The curative factors in psychoanalysis. *International Journal of Psycho-analysis* 43:194–205.

Glover, E. 1931. The therapeutic effect of inexact interpretation. In *The Technique of Psycho-Analysis.* New York: International Universities Press.

Glover, E. 1955. *The Technique of Psycho-Analysis.* New York: International Universities Press.

Goodman, N. 1984. *Of Mind and Other Matters*. Cambridge, Mass.: Harvard University Press.

Gordon, L. 1988. *Eliot's New Life*. New York: Farrar, Straus and Giroux.

Gould, S. 1977. *Ontogeny and Phylogeny*. Cambridge, Mass.: Harvard University Press.

Green, A. 1975. The analyst, symbolization and absence in the analytic setting. *International Journal of Psycho-analysis* 56:1–22.

Greenacre, P. 1953. The predisposition to anxiety, Part I and Part II. In *Trauma, Growth and Personality*. London: Hogarth Press.

—— 1954. The role of transference: Practical considerations in relation to psychoanalytic therapy. *Journal of the American Psychoanalytic Association* 2:671–684.

Greenson, R. 1967. *The Technique and Practice of Psychoanalysis*. New York: International Universities Press.

Greenson, R., and M. Wexler. 1969. The non-transference relationship in the psychoanalytic situation. *International Journal of Psycho-analysis* 50:27–40.

—— 1970. Discussion of the non-transference relationship in the psychoanalytic situation. *International Journal of Psycho-analysis* 51:143–145.

Gross, A. 1949. Sense of time in dreams. *Psychoanalytic Quarterly* 8:466–470.

Hearne, V. 1986. *Adam's Task*. New York: Knopf.

Heimann, P. 1950. On counter-transference. *International Journal of Psycho-analysis* 31:81–84.

Hoffer, A. 1985. Toward a definition of psychoanalytic neutrality. *Journal of the American Psychoanalytic Association* 33:771–795.

Holton, G. 1973. The roots of complementarity. In *Thematic Origins of Scientific Thought*. Cambridge, Mass.: Harvard University Press.

Huizinga, J. 1955. *Homo Ludens*. Boston: Beacon Press.

Jackson, S. 1969. The history of Freud's concepts of regression. *Journal of the American Psychoanalytic Association* 17:743–784.

James, W. 1890. *The Principles of Psychology*, vol. 1. New York: Dover, 1950.

Jaques, E. 1982. *The Form of Time*. London: Heinemann.

Joffe, W., and J. Sandler. 1965. Notes on pain, depression, and individuation. *Psychoanalytic Study of the Child* 20:394–424.

Jones, E. 1953. *The Life and Work of Sigmund Freud,* vol. 1. New York: Basic Books.

Kafka, J. 1964. Technical applications of a concept of multiple reality. *International Journal of Psycho-analysis* 45:575–578.

—— 1977. On reality: An examination of object constancy, ambiguity, paradox and time. In *Thought, Consciousness and Reality,* ed. J. Smith. New Haven: Yale University Press.

Kagan, J., S. Reznick, and N. Snidman. 1988. Biological bases of childhood shyness. *Science* 240:167–171.

Kermode, F. 1985. Freud and interpretation. *International Review of Psycho-analysis* 12:3–12.

King, P. 1962. Discussion: Curative factors in psycho-analysis. *International Journal of Psycho-analysis* 53:225–227.

Klauber, J. 1981. *Difficulties in the Analytic Encounter.* New York: Jason Aronson.

—— 1982. The role of illusion in the psychoanalytic cure. (Unpublished paper.)

Klein, M. 1963. *Our Adult World.* New York: Basic Books.

Kohut, H. 1977. *The Restoration of the Self.* New York: International Universities Press.

—— 1984. *How Does Analysis Cure?* Chicago: University of Chicago Press.

Kris, A. 1977. Either-or dilemmas. *Psychoanalytic Study of the Child* 32:91–117.

—— 1985. Resistance in convergent and divergent conflicts. *Psychoanalytic Quarterly* 54:537–568.

Kumin, I. 1978. Developmental aspects of opposites and paradox. *International Review of Psycho-analysis* 5:477–483.

Kundera, M. 1984. *The Unbearable Lightness of Being.* New York: Harper.

Lacan, J. 1978. *The Four Fundamental Concepts of Psycho-Analysis.* New York: Norton.

Laplanche, J., and J. B. Pontalis. 1973. *The Language of Psychoanalysis.* New York: Norton.

Leach, E. 1986. The big fish in the biblical wilderness. *International Review of Psycho-analysis* 13:129–141.

Leavy, S. 1973. Psychoanalytic interpretation. *Psychoanalytic Study of the Child* 28:305–330.

—— 1980. *The Psychoanalytic Dialogue.* New Haven: Yale University Press.

Levenson, E. 1988. Show and tell: The recursive order of transference. In *The Therapeutic Action of Psychoanalytic Psychotherapy,* ed. A. Rothstein. Madison: International Universities Press.

Lichtenstein, H. 1963. The dilemma of human identity: Notes on self-transformation, self-objectivation, and metamorphosis. *Journal of the American Psychoanalytic Association* 11:173–223.

Lipton, S. 1977. The advantages of Freud's technique as shown in his analysis of the Rat Man. *International Journal of Psycho-analysis* 58:255–274.

Little, M. 1985. Winnicott working in areas where psychotic anxieties predominate. *Free Associations* 3:9–42.

Loewald, H. 1962. Superego and time. In *Papers on Psycho-analysis.* New Haven: Yale University Press.

——— 1980. Psychoanalysis as an art and the fantasy character of the psychoanalytic situation. In *Papers on Psycho-analysis.* New Haven: Yale University Press.

——— 1981. Regression: Some general considerations. *Psychoanalytic Quarterly* 50:22–43.

London, N. 1987. Discussion. In defense of the transference neurosis concept: A process and interactional definition. *Psychoanalytic Inquiry* 7:587–598.

Macalpine, I. 1950. The development of the transference. *Psychoanalytic Quarterly* 19:501–539.

Masson, J., trans. and ed. 1985. *The Complete Letters of Sigmund Freud to Wilhelm Fliess.* Cambridge, Mass.: Harvard University Press.

Mayr, E. 1982. *The Growth of Biological Thought.* Cambridge, Mass.: Harvard University Press.

McDougall, J. 1980. *Plea for a Measure of Abnormality.* New York: International Universities Press.

——— 1985. *Theaters of the Mind.* New York: Basic Books.

Meissner, W. 1988. *Treatment of Patients in the Borderline Spectrum.* New York: Jason Aronson.

Meltzer, D. 1967. *The Psycho-Analytical Process.* Perthshire, England: Clunie Press.

Milner, M. 1955. The role of illusion in symbol formation. In *New Directions in Psychoanalysis.* New York: Basic Books.

Mitchell, S. 1988. *Relational Concepts in Psychoanalysis.* Cambridge, Mass.: Harvard University Press.

Modell, A. 1968. *Object Love and Reality.* New York: International Universities Press.

——— 1975. A narcissistic defense against affects and the illusion of self-sufficiency. *International Journal of Psycho-analysis* 56: 275–282.

——— 1975a. The ego and the id: Fifty years later. *International Journal of Psycho-analysis* 56:57–68.

——— 1976. "The holding environment" and the therapeutic action of psychoanalysis. *Journal of the American Psychoanalytic Association* 24:285–307.

——— 1984. Interpretation and symbolic actualizations of developmental arrests. In *Psychoanalyis in a New Context*. New York: International Universities Press.

——— 1984a. *Psychoanalysis in a New Context*. New York: International Universities Press.

——— 1984b. Self psychology as a psychology of conflict: Comments on the psychoanalysis of the narcissistic personality. In *Psychoanalysis: The Vital Issues*, vol. 2, ed. G. Pollock and J. Gedo. New York: International Universities Press.

——— 1985. Object relations theory. In *Models of the Mind*, ed. A. Rothstein. New York: International Universities Press.

——— 1985a. The works of Winnicott and the evolution of his thought. *Journal of the American Psychoanalytic Association* 33 (supplement):113–137.

——— 1985b. Self preservation and the preservation of the self. *Annual of Psychoanalysis* 12/13:69–86.

——— 1988. On the mode of therapeutic action of psychoanalytic therapy: Or how does treatment help? In *The Therapeutic Action of Psychoanalytic Psychotherapy*, ed. A. Rothstein. Madison, Wis.: International Universities Press.

——— 1988a. The persistence of transitional relatedness. In *The Solace Paradigm*, ed. P. Horton, H. Gewitz, and K. Kreutter. Madison: International Universities Press.

——— 1988b. The centrality of the psychoanalytic setting and the changing aims of treatment: A perspective from a theory of object relations. *Psychoanalytic Quarterly* 57:577–596.

——— 1989. The psychoanalytic setting as a container of multiple levels of reality: A perspective on the theory of psychoanalytic treatment. *Psychoanalytic Inquiry* 9:67–87.

Morgenthau, H., and E. Person. 1978. The roots of narcissism. *Partisian Review* 45:337–347.

Namnum, A. 1972. Time in psychoanalytic technique. *Journal of the American Psychoanalytic Association* 20:736–750.

Newman, K. 1984. The capacity to use the object. In *Psychoanalysis: The Vital Issues,* vol. 2, ed. G. Pollock and J. Gedo. New York: International Universities Press.

O'Flaherty, W. 1984. *Dreams, Illusions and Other Realities.* Chicago: University of Chicago Press.

Ogden, T. 1985. On potential space. *International Journal of Psychoanalysis* 66:129–141.

Orgel, S. 1965. On time and timelessness. *Journal of the American Psychoanalytic Association* 13:102–121.

Panel. 1937. Symposium of the theory of the therapeutic results of psycho-analysis. *International Journal of Psycho-analysis* 18: parts 2 and 3.

Panel. 1983. Interpretation: Toward a contemporary understanding of the term. *Journal of the American Psychoanalytic Association* 31:237–245.

Panel. 1987. Transference neurosis evolution or obsolescence. *Psychoanalytic Inquiry* 7:457–603.

Parsons, M. 1986. Suddenly finding it matters: Paradox of analyst's non-attachment. *International Journal of Psycho-analysis* 67: 475–488.

Piaget, J. 1954. *The Construction of Reality in the Child.* New York: Basic Books.

Pine, F. 1988. On the four psychologies of psychoanalysis and the nature of the therapeutic impact. In *How Does Treatment Help?,* ed. A. Rothstein. Madison, Wis.: International Universities Press.

Poland, W. 1984. On the analyst's neutrality. *Journal of the American Psychoanalytic Association* 32:283–299.

Pontalis, J. -B. 1981. Between the dream as object and the dream text. In *Frontiers in Psychoanalysis.* New York: International Universities Press.

Porder, M. 1987. Projective identification: An alternative hypothesis. *Psychoanalytic Quarterly* 56:431–451.

Proust, M. 1928. *Swan's Way.* New York: Random House Modern Library, 1956.

Racker, H. 1968. *Transference and Countertransference.* New York: International Universities Press.

Rangell, L. 1983. Defense and resistance in psychoanalysis and life. *Journal of the American Psychoanalytic Association* 31 (supplement):147–174.

Rank, O. 1936. *Truth and Reality.* New York: Norton, 1978.

Reed, G. 1987. Scientific and polemical aspects of the term. *Psychoanalytic Inquiry* 7:465–483.

Reich, W. 1949. *Character Analysis.* New York: Orgone Institute Press.

Richards, I. 1969. *Coleridge on Imagination.* Bloomington: Indiana University Press.

Ricoeur, P. 1970. *Freud and Philosophy,* trans. D. Savage. New Haven: Yale University Press.

——— 1984. *Time and Narrative,* trans. K. McLaughlin. Chicago: University of Chicago Press.

Rosenfeld, I. 1988. *The Invention of Memory.* New York: Basic Books.

Rothenberg, A. 1988. *The Creative Process of Psychotherapy.* New York: Norton.

Russell, P. 1985. The structure and function of paradox in the treatment process. (Unpublished paper.)

Rycroft, C. 1985. *Psycho-Analysis and Beyond.* London: Chatto and Windus.

Sandler, J. 1960. The background of safety. *International Journal of Psycho-analysis* 41:352–356.

——— 1987. The concept of projective identification. In *Projection, Identification, Projective Identification,* ed. J. Sandler. New York: International Universities Press.

Schafer, R. 1981. *Narrative Actions in Psychoanalysis.* Worcester, Mass.: Clark University Press.

——— 1983. *The Analytic Attitude.* New York: Basic Books.

——— 1985. Wild analysis. *Journal of the American Psychoanalytic Association* 33:275–299.

Schiffer, I. 1978. *The Trauma of Time.* New York: International Universities Press.

Schwaber, E. 1983. Psychoanalytic listening and psychic reality. *International Review of Psycho-analysis* 10:379–392.

Sechehaye, M. 1951. *Symbolic Realization.* New York: International Universities Press.

Segal, H. 1981. *Melanie Klein.* New York: Penguin Books.

Sherwood, M. 1969. *The Logic of Explanation in Psychoanalysis.* New York: Academic Press.

Slavin, M. 1985. The origins of psychic conflict and the adaptive function of repression: An evolutionary biological view. *Psychoanalysis and Contemporary Thought* 8:407–440.

Spence, D. 1982. *Narrative Truth and Historical Truth*. New York: Basic Books.

Spender, S. 1986. On fame and the writer. *New York Review of Books* 33 (20):75.

Spitz, R. 1956. Countertransference: Comments on its varying role in the psychoanalytic situation. *Journal of the American Psychoanalytic Association* 4:256–265.

Spruiell, V. 1983. The rules and frames of the psychoanalytic situation. *Psychoanalytic Quarterly* 52:1–33.

Sterba, R. 1934. The fate of the ego in analytic therapy. *International Journal of Psycho-analysis* 15:117–126.

Stern, D. 1985. *The Interpersonal World of the Infant*. New York: Basic Books.

Stone, L. 1961. *The Psychoanalytic Situation*. New York: International Universities Press.

———— 1967. The psychoanalytic situation and transference: Postscript to an earlier communication. *Journal of the American Psychoanalytic Association* 15:3–58.

Strachey, J. 1934. The nature of the therapeutic action of psychoanalysis (reprinted). *International Journal of Psycho-analysis* 50: 275–292, 1969.

Sullivan, H. 1950. The illusion of personal individuality. *Psychiatry* 13:317–332.

Sulloway, F. 1979. *Freud: Biologist of the Mind*. New York: Basic Books.

Thomä, H. 1989. Freud's concept of *Nachträglichkeit* and its translation. Paper given at the Symposium on Translation and Transition, London, April 20–22, 1989.

Thomä, H., and H. Kächele. 1987. *Psychoanalytic Practice*. Berlin: Springer-Verlag.

Treurniet, N. 1980. On the relation between concepts of the self and ego in Kohut's psychology of the self. *International Journal of Psycho-analysis* 61:325–333.

Trivers, R. 1985. *Social Evolution*. Menlo Park, Calif.: Benjamin/Cummings.

Valenstein, A. 1973. On attachment to painful feelings and the negative therapeutic reaction. *Psychoanalytic Study of the Child* 28: 365–392.

———— 1979. The concept of "classical" analysis. *Journal of the American Psychoanalytic Association* 27 (supplement):113–136.

Viderman, S. 1979. The analytic space: Meaning and problems. *Psychoanalytic Quarterly* 48:257–291.

Vygotsky, L. 1986. *Thought and Language,* ed. A. Kozulin. Cambridge, Mass.: MIT Press.

Wachtel, P. 1980. The relevance of Piaget to the psychoanalytic theory of transference. *Annual of Psychoanalysis* 8:59–76. New York: International Universities Press.

Wallerstein, R. 1983. Self-psychology and "classical" psychoanalytic psychology: The nature of their relationship—a review and overview. In *The Future of Psychoanalysis,* ed. A. Goldberg. New York: International Universities Press.

Watzlawick, P., ed. 1984. *The Invented Reality.* New York: Norton.

Watzlawick, P., J. Bavelas, and D. Jackson. 1967. *Pragmatics of Human Communication.* New York: Norton.

Weiss, J., and H. Sampson. 1986. *The Psychoanalytic Process.* New York: Guilford Press.

Werman, D. 1977. Normal and pathological nostalgia. *Journal of the American Psychoanalytic Association* 25:387–398.

Winnicott, D. W. 1954. Metapsychological and clinical aspects of regression within the psycho-analytical set-up. In *Collected Papers.* New York: Basic Books, 1958.

———— 1958. *Collected Papers.* New York: Basic Books.

———— 1958a. The capacity to be alone. In *The Maturational Processes and the Facilitating Environment.* New York: International Universities Press, 1965.

———— 1963. The development of the capacity for concern. In *The Maturational Processes and the Facilitating Environment.* New York: International Universities Press, 1965.

———— 1969. The use of an object and relating through identifications. In *Playing and Reality.* New York: Basic Books, 1971.

———— 1971. Mirror-role of mother and family in child development. In *Playing and Reality.* New York: Basic Books.

———— 1975. *Through Paediatrics to Psycho-Analysis.* Introduction by M. Khan. London: Hogarth Press.

———— 1986. *Holding and Interpretation.* New York: Grove Press.

———— 1988. *Human Nature.* New York: Schocken.

Wittgenstein, L. 1984. *Culture and Value,* trans. P. Winch. Chicago: University of Chicago Press.

Wolff, P. 1988. The real and reconstructed past. *Psychoanalysis and Contemporary Thought* 11:379–414.

Wollheim, R. 1984. *The Thread of Life*. Cambridge, Mass.: Harvard University Press.

Zetzel, E. 1949. Anxiety and the capacity to bear it. In *The Capacity for Emotional Growth*. New York: International Universities Press, 1970.

―――― 1956. An approach to the relation between concept and content in psychoanalytic theory: With special reference to the work of Melanie Klein and her followers. *Psychoanalytic Study of the Child* 11:99–121.

―――― 1958. Therapeutic alliance in the analysis of hysteria. In *The Capacity for Emotional Growth*. New York: International Universities Press, 1970.

―――― 1970. *The Capacity for Emotional Growth*. New York: International Universities Press.

Index